ADVANCE
Awakening: Asp
through Integral Yoga

Awakening: Aspiration to Realization through Integral Yoga is a carefully crafted set of stories and teachings about the deeper practice of Yoga that makes this profound subject alive and relevant for everyone. The book is refreshing, insightful and indicative of the higher essence of Yoga. Notably, *Awakening* reflects the enduring inspiration of Swami Satchidananda, one of the master Gurus who brought Yoga to the West. The author, Swami Karunananda, understands body, mind, and deeper consciousness and can guide the reader in the soul's journey of integral Self-discovery.

—David Frawley (Vamadeva Shastri), author of *Vedic Yoga: The Path of the Rishi*, founder and director of the American Institute of Vedic Studies

Awakening is a reflection of the essence and heart of Sri Gurudev Swami Satchidananda's teachings of Integral Yoga. Its poetic narrative takes us on the journey of transformation, drawing upon the ancient wisdom of Yoga as well as the inspirational stories and sayings of masters from many interfaith traditions. It weaves a tapestry of varying paths of Yoga and how they can be applied and integrated into every aspect of our lives in the world of today. *Awakening* is a timeless reminder that Yoga is not just a physical practice but also the soul's longing for the remembrance of the Divine in the union that is Yoga.

—Rama Jyoti Vernon, author of *Yoga: The Practice of Myth and Sacred Geometry*; founder, California Yoga Teachers Association; co-founder, *Yoga Journal*

Swami Karunananda has written a magnificent book in honor of the 100th birth anniversary of Sri Swami Satchidananda. *Awakening* is a fresh, insightful, and timely examination of the wisdom tradition of Yoga—aimed directly at the heart of the particular suffering of our time. Swami Karunananda takes a highly integrative approach, relating the wisdom of Yoga to other major spiritual traditions. This is an inspiring work that every contemporary yogi will want to have in his or her library.

—Stephen Cope, director, Kripalu Institute for Extraordinary Living; author of *The Wisdom of Yoga: A Seeker's Guide to Extraordinary Living* and *The Great Work of Your Life: A Guide for the Journey to Your True Calling*

An eclectic collection of insights and reflections on the spiritual life from a lifelong practitioner and senior disciple of Swami Satchidananda, drawing on anecdotes and teachings from various wisdom traditions of the world. There are inspirations to be found on every page for the sincere spiritual seeker.

—Edwin Bryant, author of *The Yoga Sutras of Patanjali: A New Edition, Translation, and Commentary* and professor of Hinduism, Rutgers University

This is a book, grounded in faith, that can change the way you see yourself and offer you a direct path to God-realization. The philosophy, practices, and inspiring stories from spiritual masters in many traditions weave through the author's own self-revealing journey to "peace, happiness and freedom," and offer a blueprint for personal and global transformation. From the depths of her studies with and transmission from the master yogi, Sri Swami Satchidananda, and a lifetime of contemplative practice, Swami Karunananda offers a blueprint for living a Self-realized life in the midst of the common heartaches of our daily existence.

—Amy Weintraub, MFA, E-RYT500, author of *Yoga Skills for Therapists, Yoga for Depression*, and founding director, LifeForce Yoga Healing Institute

Awakening: Aspiration to Realization through Integral Yoga is a compelling, empowering and practical guide to realizing freedom in this very lifetime. This comprehensive and accessible book, filled with profound stories that inspire and illuminate, is a perfect companion on the path to realization.

—Matthew Flickstein, author of *The Meditator's Workbook, The Meditator's Atlas, Voices of Truth*, and founder of The Forest Way Meditation Center

AWAKENING

ASPIRATION TO REALIZATION
THROUGH INTEGRAL YOGA

SWAMI KARUNANANDA

Beloved Rebecca,
  ॐ May your life and path
be filled with blessings in
abundance — all health, happiness,
peace & spiritual awakening —

  With Love & Prayers
  Swami Karun ॐ

Other Titles Available from Integral Yoga® Publications

Books by Sri Swami Satchidananda

Adversity and Awakening
Beyond Words
The Breath of Life
Free Yourself
Gems of Wisdom
The Golden Present
The Healthy Vegetarian
Heaven on Earth
Integral Yoga Hatha

Kailash Journal
The Key to Peace
To Know Your Self
The Living Gita
Meditation
Overcoming Obstacles
Pathways to Peace
Satchidananda Sutras
The Yoga Sutras of Patanjali

Books from Other Authors

Bound to Be Free: The Liberating Power of Prison Yoga
by Rev. Sandra Kumari de Sachy, Ed.D.

Enlightening Tales As Told By Sri Swami Satchidananda
edited by Swami Karunananda

Hatha Yoga for Kids by Kids by the Children of Yogaville

Inside the Yoga Sutras by Rev. Jaganath Carrera

Lotus Prayer Book edited by Swami Karunananda

Sparkling Together by Jyoti Ma

A Vision of Peace: The Interfaith Teachings of Sri Swami Satchidananda
by Rev. Sandra Kumari de Sachy, Ed.D.

ISBN 978-1-938477-17-1

Printed in the United States of America on recycled text stock.

Integral Yoga® Publications, Satchidananda Ashram–Yogaville®, Inc.
108 Yogaville Way, Buckingham, Virginia, USA 23921
www.Yogaville.org

AWAKENING

ASPIRATION TO REALIZATION THROUGH INTEGRAL YOGA

SWAMI KARUNANANDA

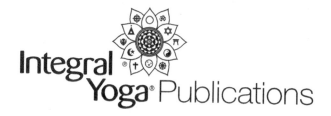

Integral Yoga® Publications

Buckingham, Virginia

Dedication

Lovingly offered in honor of
the 100th Birth Anniversary of
His Holiness Sri Swami Satchidananda

With deepest reverence and gratitude
for his teachings and guidance
that awaken the Spirit and transform lives

CONTENTS

FOREWORD

It's not every day that I get the opportunity to assist in the compilation of a book of teachings that transforms lives. Such is the power of the Integral Yoga teachings of Sri Swami Satchidananda (Sri Gurudev), one of the world's great Yoga masters; and that power and those teachings are reflected in the writings of Swami Karunananda, a senior disciple of Sri Gurudev and herself a beloved teacher. When Swami Karunananda mentioned that she was considering putting together a collection of essays as an offering for the centennial celebration of Sri Gurudev's 100th birth anniversary, I quickly offered to serve in any way that might be of assistance. I know the power of these teachings to help us experience more peace, joy, and meaning in our lives.

Before discovering Integral Yoga in 2003, I was a stressed out attorney practicing law. I also practiced many bad habits, including drinking and smoking. I weighed well over 200 pounds and my knees hurt when I walked. I was successful in my professional life, but inwardly miserable.

I first heard Sri Gurudev speak in July 2002 at Satchidananda Ashram–Yogaville in Virginia. It was one of his last *satsangs*, and I was struck by his wisdom. Afterward, I continued to live as I had been, but began to grow more aware of how unhappy and unhealthy I was.

I returned to the *ashram* in 2003 for a weekend stress management workshop. Dr. Amrita McLanahan, another senior disciple of Sri Gurudev, spoke about the human condition and the way to end suffering. I began to see life differently, realizing that my life did not have to be the way it was. Dr. McLanahan's prescription for me included changing to a vegetarian diet, doing Hatha Yoga and meditation every day, and quitting smoking and drinking. She also recommended Sri Gurudev's book, *To Know Your Self.*

Before I left the *ashram* that weekend, I was at the entrance to the road leading to LOTUS, the beautiful interfaith shrine, when I had an intense experience of total knowing and reassurance that everything was going to be all right; I didn't have to worry about anything anymore. This profound sense of peace continued for a few days.

My life has not been the same ever since that day in Yogaville. I began putting Sri Gurudev's teachings into practice and immediately began experiencing the benefits. I lost 60 pounds within one year. My body stopped aching. My spirit was lighter. I haven't had or desired a drink or a cigarette since that day. While I'm certainly not perfect, I'm healthier and happier. I continue to practice law, but I haven't looked at that, or anything else, in quite the same way. Yoga has become a lens through which I see life. I think more about how my life and work fit within the larger picture, and how I can best serve others in the interconnected world in which we live.

I fell in love with Sri Gurudev's Integral Yoga teachings, and those teachings, practices, and the Integral Yoga community have been woven into the fabric of my life. I have become certified to teach Integral Yoga Hatha and Raja Yoga. Desiring to go deeper spiritually, I received mantra initiation. When I had the opportunity to live and serve at Yogaville in 2012, I didn't hesitate. It gave me a chance to learn and grow in a Yoga community, immersed in the teachings and lifestyle.

One of the blessings of having a spiritual master is that the master's teachings never die. The teachings and their transformative power live on in so many ways, including through the teaching and service of senior disciples. As I have continued to learn and practice more in the Integral Yoga tradition, Swami Karunananda's teachings have become a treasured part of my spiritual curriculum. Soon after my Yogaville experience in 2003, I discovered her articles in *Integral Yoga Magazine*. When each new issue arrived, I eagerly turned the pages to find her featured article. Her articles always seemed tailor-made for me, speaking to the very questions that were on my mind and heart.

I am so pleased that *Awakening: Aspiration to Realization through Integral Yoga* is available for all those who seek more knowledge of Yoga and its deeper meaning. The book addresses topics ranging from formal Yoga practice to applying Yoga off the mat in daily life. It clearly explains the philosophy of Yoga and includes some personal experiences of Swami Karunananda that transformed her life. Faith, fear, attachment, obstacles, forgiveness, healing, suffering, and transformation are among the topics that Swami Karunananda addresses as she offers guidance on how to progress on the spiritual path. *Awakening* speaks to the depths of my heart.

Swami Karunananda's writings offer tools with which to deal with these challenging times. During an era marked by climate change, economic tension, political paralysis, war, and violence, many are seeking answers to the age-old questions of who we are and why we are here—and how we can live differently, with greater peace and happiness. Integral Yoga provides answers to those questions and offers a road map to guide us along the journey of life. It is a comprehensive system aimed at developing all aspects of the individual—physical, mental, emotional, and spiritual—providing opportunities for growth, transformation, and the experience of inner peace.

Swami Karunananda is my beloved mentor and teacher. I cannot adequately express the great joy and privilege it has been for me to assist Swami Karunananda in seeing this book to fruition. She conveys the Integral Yoga teachings with keen intellect, remarkable spiritual insight, and a heart full of compassion. She has been such a blessing to me on my spiritual path and my gratitude to her is beyond words.

Montina Sraddha Cole
Co-founder of EduSeed, a nonprofit promoting education among underserved communities
April 3, 2014

PREFACE

Sri Swami Satchidananda is my spiritual Guru. Meeting him in 1970 changed my life. My mind was opened to new possibilities, my heart discovered new ways to love and care for others, my life found new meaning and direction. My gratitude is boundless.

The year 2014 marks the 100th anniversary of his birth. I wanted to make an offering as a token of my love and reverence. So, the idea came to compile the articles I had written for *Integral Yoga Magazine* from 2002 – 2012 into a book. The articles contained his teachings as I understood and had practiced them for over forty years, along with stories about him and the Integral Yoga Institutes.

That's how the project began. It quickly took on a life of its own and became much more.

The articles changed and expanded; new ones were written. My understanding deepened. It has been a journey that has culminated in the current volume. There is some repetition of key concepts and practices, since the articles spanned a decade. Swami Sivananda, who was Swami Satchidananda's Guru, was a prolific writer. He said such repetition was good; it helped us to remember the points.

For those who were around when Yoga first began to take root in the West, I hope the recollections shared rekindle your own cherished memories of early days on the path. For younger generations who are just discovering Yoga, I hope this collection conveys the dedication and commitment that enabled Yoga to grow from humble beginnings to a global phenomenon.

Yoga as we know it today is the result of the vision of great masters, their tireless transmission of the teachings, and the efforts of thousands upon thousands of Yoga practitioners who took those teachings to heart and put them into practice.

And the journey continues with each new person who does their first *asana*, with each sincere seeker who sits for meditation, with each dynamic yogi who dedicates time and energy in serving others. As, one by one, people awaken to their own higher potential and discover the abiding peace within their own hearts, we will become that much closer to living in a world established in peace and filled with loving-kindness. That is the beauty and the gift that Yoga has to offer.

Swami Karunananda
Satchidananda Ashram–Yogaville
April 19, 2014

ACKNOWLEDGMENTS

It takes a village to raise a child, and it takes a team to produce a book. This book was brought to fruition through the efforts of a wonderful and talented group of people who I am blessed to call my friends. My humble and profound thanks goes to:

Montina Sraddha Cole who compiled, organized, and analyzed all the articles I had written for the *Integral Yoga® Magazine*, as well as reviewed new material as it was produced. Thanks to her prodigious efforts and careful research, we also have a wonderful glossary for the book.

Swami Sarvaananda, Ph.D. who was an enthusiastic and insightful reader of everything I wrote, providing valuable feedback and support every step of the way.

Gerald Satyam Penn, Professor of Computer Science at the University of Toronto, and Rev. Paraman Barsel who reviewed the more philosophical articles in this collection. The depth and subtlety of their understanding were an invaluable resource.

Satyam Penn and Rev. Lakshmi Barsel, Ph.D. for their expert guidance in transliterating all the Sanskrit words and phrases in the text.

Karuna Kreps for her skillful copyediting, Swami Hamsananda for her careful proofreading, and Shiva Herve for his patient layout of the book.

Sherry Gayatri Van Dyke for the beautiful cover artwork.

Rev. Prem Anjali, Ph.D. whose one-pointed dedication to the dissemination of the teachings of Integral Yoga made the publication of this book possible. When she offered many months prior to serve as Project Manager, I had no idea what that would entail. Suffice it to say, she set the course and brought us to the finish line.

Thank you to all my dear friends and to so many well-respected teachers in the Yoga community for all the prayers and blessings— your good wishes and support have meant the world to me.

We would also like to express our deep gratitude to the Harry and Padma Wadhwani family and the Chandru and Laxmi Wadhwani family for their generous donations in support of the Global Garland projects in honor of the 100th Birth Anniversary of His Holiness Sri Swami Satchidananda.

We also thank the following for their permission to quote:

Excerpts of Brother Lawrence's writings from *The Practice of the Presence of God*. Translated by Robert J. Edmonson. Edited by Hal M. Helms, © 2010. Reprinted with permission of Paraclete Press.

Excerpt of Hafiz poem from *I Heard God Laughing: Renderings of Hafiz* by Daniel Ladinsky, © 1996. Reprinted with permission.

Excerpt of Li Po poem, from *With Beauty Before Me* by Joseph Cornell, © 2000. Reprinted with permission.

Excerpts from *Tao Teh Ching*, translated by John C. H. Wu, © 1961 by St. John's University Press, New York. Reprinted by arrangement with The Permissions Company, Inc., on behalf of Shambhala Publications, Inc., Boston, www.shambhala.com.

INTRODUCTION

Vision and Legacy

There's a story about a man who was strolling through the countryside, when, suddenly, he fell into a large, gaping hole. After a while, someone passed by, and the man eagerly called out, "Please help me, I'm down here in the hole." The passerby, being a doctor, replied, "Yes, I see your predicament." He wrote a prescription, tossed it into the hole, and proceeded on his way. Next, an engineer came by. The man repeated his fervent cry. The engineer assured him, "I can certainly help you, but I will need a contract and an advance for my costs." The man called out, "But I'm down here in the hole; I can't provide that right now." The engineer expressed his regrets and walked on. Then, a theologian came upon the scene. He determined it was necessary to consult scripture and said he would get back to the man after a thorough examination of the situation.

Finally, a holy sage appeared. Despairing now, the man called out, "Can you please help me? I'm down here in the hole." Without any hesitation, the holy man jumped into the hole. Confused and somewhat annoyed, the man looked at him and said, "What have you accomplished? Now, there are two of us in the hole." "Yes," replied the sage, "but I have been here before, and I know the way out."

Spiritual masters who have experienced the supreme truth, who embody the peace and joy of the Divine, know the way out of the pain and uncertainty that are common to human existence. From the vantage of the Absolute, filled with the vision of the universal Spirit, they are able to reach out to sincere seekers and provide a map, a guidebook, to freedom.

Sri Swami Satchidananda, sometimes referred to as Sri Gurudev, was one of the great Yoga masters who came to the West from India in the 1960s. He founded and continues to be the spiritual inspiration for the Integral Yoga organization. While rooted in universal consciousness, he understood his students' aspirations and limitations. He knew the path and how to successfully navigate the journey. He found a way to package and deliver the yogic teachings that not only engaged our attention, but also enabled us to practice. Like a step-down transformer, he converted the universal into the particular; he translated the power of the ineffable into a form that could be utilized by the individual on a regular, daily basis, resulting in profound transformation.

Sri Gurudev straddled both realities—what Adi Shankaracharya referred to as *paramarthika sat* and *laukika sat*: absolute and relative reality. At a memorable *satsang*, he described this state of dual awareness and announced that it was the *samadhi* for Integral Yogis. Known as *sahaja samadhi*, which translates as "the easy, natural *samadhi*," it entails simultaneously experiencing the unity underlying all creation and the diversity of the myriad names and forms—like being at the very depth of the ocean where it is always calm and, at the same time, on the surface with all the waves, bubbles, foam, and spray. Firmly established in the unity, you could skillfully interact with the diversity. Exquisitely, he exemplified and modeled this for all of us.

Abiding in the highest consciousness, he was always completely present in the moment and his very presence quickened, awakened, the Spirit within us. One of the greatest teaching moments I experienced was not hearing him expound on the scriptures, or taking a Hatha Yoga class from him, or even receiving personal guidance. It occurred during a Yoga retreat in Santa Barbara. I was serving as the coordinator and my mind was overly busy, filled with a plethora of details.

I simply had to hand Gurudev a piece of paper with information. My mind was jumping all over, already planning its next task. As I leaned forward to give him the paper, he gently, consciously extended his hand to receive it, totally focused on that particular interaction. At that moment, it seemed like I was all that existed for him and receiving that paper was all that mattered. The incessant whirling of my mind stopped; for an instant, everything stood still. I experienced perfect peace.

Being aware of our diverse temperaments and backgrounds, he presented the teachings in a way that people from all faiths and traditions could embrace. He prepared an abundant feast, and all were welcome to dine at his table. Once at a *satsang*, I recall looking around the room and noting that, in this simple hall in rural Virginia, there were guests from every continent, except Antarctica!

Sri Gurudev began his life as a Hindu, born into an orthodox family. But at some point on his journey, he decided to become an "Undo." He explained that originally we were *fine*, but we had become *defined* by our attachments and false identifications, and all that we needed to do was to *refine* ourselves to realize our true nature. Seeing all the problems in the world perpetrated in the name of religion, his boundless spirit couldn't be confined to a particular designation. Once he quipped that if he were put in charge of the world for a day, he would know how to restore peace. He would put all the politicians in one boat and all the religious leaders in another. He would send both boats out to sea, and then everyone remaining could live peacefully together.

His life, his teachings, his mission were all about peace—peace for the individual and peace for the world. For the individual, he imparted the teachings of Integral Yoga, a synthesis of the six main branches of Yoga—Raja, Hatha, Karma, Bhakti, Jnana, and Japa—that addresses every aspect of life and provides for the harmonious development of every level of the individual: physical, mental, emotional, intellectual, social, and spiritual. While presenting specific precepts and practices for his students, his all-embracing spirit also described Yoga as encompassing anything that would enable one to be easeful, peaceful, and useful. The past decades have seen these teachings transform the lives of thousands of seekers, as well as help to revolutionize the health care profession, as the Integral Yoga approach has been incorporated into the treatment for heart disease, cancer, and other ailments.

On the global level, Sri Gurudev's mission of peace focused on promoting interfaith dialogue and understanding. In 1986, on a trip sponsored by the Center for Soviet-American Dialogue (later named the Center for International Dialogue), he was meeting in Moscow with members of the Russian clergy. After some time, his translator became annoyed with all the talk about God and started challenging him. "We don't believe in that," she said, "we are nonbelievers." Sri Gurudev calmly replied, "There's nothing wrong in that, but could you please tell me what is it that you do not believe?" She didn't know what to say, so he questioned her further: "You don't believe in going to a church or a synagogue? You don't believe in reading any scriptures?" She emphatically answered, "No!" After a few more suggestions about what she did not believe in, he gently asked: "But don't you believe in friendship? In loving people? In comradeship?" "Yes, we do!" she happily stated. "So, you do have something you believe. Then how can you call yourself a nonbeliever? What you believe is the real religion. Religion should educate us to love everyone equally, to have universal friendship, universal comradeship. You believe in the fundamental truths behind all the religions, so you should not call yourself a nonbeliever."

In the same year, he dedicated LOTUS, the Light Of Truth Universal Shrine. This was the fruition of a vision he had long cherished for an interfaith shrine where people of all faiths and backgrounds could come to pray and meditate together. Several years prior, with little money on hand, he performed a *puja*, mounted a bulldozer, drove out onto a large, barren field, and began excavating the site for the LOTUS lake. Addressing the concerns of his practical-minded devotees, he said, "This is God's work. If God wants it to happen, all that we need will come." And little by little, drop-by-drop, it did.

One day, there was a call from the bank informing us that an anonymous donor, inspired by the project, was wiring $108,000 into our account. From all over the globe, people came forward to participate. The outpouring of creative energy was enormous. Everyone's skills were engaged and expanded; inconceivable tasks were accomplished, as a new creation was brought into manifestation. Twenty years after Sri Gurudev first landed in New York, almost to the day, the Light Of Truth Universal Shrine (LOTUS) was inaugurated in a glorious ceremony that drew clergy and dignitaries from all over the globe.

Bold red letters across the main archway leading to the shrine proclaim, "Truth is One, Paths are Many," Sri Gurudev's rendering of the ancient *Vedic* saying: "*Ekam sat viprah bahudha vadanti.*" This means: "Truth is one; seers express it in many ways," reminding us to remember the unity underlying all the faiths, while respecting and enjoying their diversity. Around a central light are ten altars representing the world's major faiths, including altars to the Native American and African faiths. There are also symbols to represent all other known faiths and even unknown ones, those yet to come or the private paths of individuals. In the All Faiths Hall below, there's even a display called "Secular Faiths" for those who seek the truth or higher good through other means—like music, philosophy, science, or ecology. Sri Gurudev wanted LOTUS to be a sacred place of blessing for everyone—a beacon of universal peace and harmony.

He had the vision and courage to conduct a divine experiment. With extraordinary patience, insight, and skill he transplanted the wisdom of the East into Western soil, into an environment ripe for change that was like a plant seeking the light. His creativity, broadmindedness, and all-inclusiveness are apparent everywhere. At Yogaville, he placed a monastery in the midst of a community, encouraging everyone to practice, pray, and serve together. He established both a *Sannyas* (monastic) Order and an Integral Yoga Ministry, providing opportunities for those called to fully dedicate themselves in these ways. He designed the schedule to strike a balance between the contemplative and active life, affirming that one needn't withdraw from the world to attain spiritual goals. For educational purposes, he provided an academy for Yoga students, a school for children based on yogic principles, and a Fine Arts Society for instruction in dance and music.

Toward the end of his physical life, he lovingly confided that he had given us everything, that there was nothing he had withheld, nothing more that we needed. Now, it is up to us to move forward, honoring our roots—the lineage and legacy that have been bestowed on us—and stretching our wings, as we carry his mission and teachings into the future.

EXPLORATION

Journeying to Enlightenment

If someone were to ask, "What do you want most out of life?" chances are good that your response would be, "I want to be happy." Everyone wants to be happy; it is the underlying want behind all the other wants in life. Generally, we seek it in external ways—but, eventually, we realize that whatever we may amass or achieve is not going to bring us lasting happiness. We become disenchanted with the fleeting pleasure that comes from trying to satisfy our desires. At that point, we become spiritual seekers.

We're ready now to venture into new territory, to find fulfillment in a different way. Our exploration into other possibilities begins and we may find ourselves checking out various Yoga schools, visiting spiritual centers, or even diving deeper into our own faith traditions. The important thing to consider whenever we're about to embark on a path is: Where is it going to lead us, and how are we going to get there? The same is true when we're selecting our spiritual path.

That is where the philosophical teachings of Yoga can be very helpful. They describe the goal of Yoga—the final destination—and the practices that will get us there. As we have different temperaments and capacities, there are different branches of Yoga to guide us on the journey to spiritual awakening. Each branch of Yoga describes the goal a little differently and prescribes different practices to get there but, ultimately, they all enable us to realize that the peace and happiness we seek is our own true nature.

Integral Yoga offers a synthesis of the various branches of Yoga so that there is a harmonious development and integration of every level of the individual—social, physical, emotional, intellectual, and spiritual. There are six branches:

Raja Yoga—the path of meditation and self-discipline, based on ethical principles

Hatha Yoga—purification and strengthening of the system through *asanas* (postures), *pranayama* (breathing techniques), deep relaxation, and *kriyas* (cleansing practices)

Karma Yoga—the path of selfless service

Bhakti Yoga—the path of devotion to the Divine

Jnana Yoga—the path of wisdom, based on study, analysis, and cultivation of awareness

Japa Yoga—concentrated repetition of a mantra, mystic sounds that represent a particular aspect of the Divine

The goal of Integral Yoga is to realize the Spirit within and then to see that same Spirit in everyone and everything. This is an enlightened state of consciousness in which we recognize the spiritual unity behind all the diversity in creation. With this awareness, we can come together, work together, and live together harmoniously. It's a formula for peace in the challenging times in which we live.

Wake Up!

"Eating, drinking, sleeping! A little laughter, much weeping! Is that all? Do not die here like a worm. Wake up! Attain immortal bliss!" This is the clarion call sounded from the Himalayas by the great sage, Sri Swami Sivananda, who was the Guru of my spiritual teacher, Swami Satchidananda. The *Bhagavad Gita* proclaims: "What seems night to others is the state of awakening for one with a disciplined mind. What appears day to others is as night to the sage who knows the Self." In other words, sages abide in the true Self; that is "day" for them. From that vantage, they see the world as illusion. Other people, in general, are asleep to the state of enlightenment; their vision is limited to worldly phenomena, and that is "day" for them. The sage and the average person have opposite experiences as to what is real and what is unreal. How do these experiences compare?

Awakened: You have realized your true Self; you experience perfect peace and joy. You see the same essence in everyone and everything, the underlying reality that pervades all creation. You are established in that which is unchanging, indestructible, and everlasting; and you are free from all sorrow, fear, and delusion.

Asleep: You identify yourself as the body and mind, and feel limited and separate from others. You function on the level of duality, tossed by the pairs of opposites—like pleasure/pain, loss/gain, praise/blame—and pulled by the shifting tides of attachment and aversion. Impermanence, uncertainty, and vulnerability give rise to suffering.

Given the options, the choice seems obvious: Wake up! This is easier said than done. Throughout the ages, sages, philosophers, and mystics have pondered the dichotomy between the never-changing reality—the substratum, support, and essence of creation—and the ever-changing phenomena of ordinary experience. The different branches of Yoga, as well as the varied faith traditions, address in their own ways, these two levels of existence. They assign different terms, provide a philosophical context, and then present distinct methods to enable one to transcend the ephemeral and experience the eternal.

They explain how or why the reality is veiled from our perception, and, in so doing, present some kind of mechanism of delusion. Some systems subscribe to dualism; others take a non-dualistic approach.

Raja Yoga

The Raja Yoga that is presented in the *Yoga Sutras* is a dualistic system. Patanjali posits two eternal principles, *Purusha* and *Prakriti*. *Purusha* refers to the never-changing Self or Seer, and *Prakriti* is the ever-changing creation or nature. *Purusha* is pure consciousness; everything else is material. In our essence, we are that pure consciousness. We are the Seer, but we take ourselves to be the body, which is part of nature. We think we are the mind, which is also part of nature, comprised of subtle matter. But the mind in itself is not conscious. It stands in relation to the Self, as does the moon to the sun; the mind appears to be conscious because it reflects the light of the Self.

The purpose of *Prakriti* is to provide us with experiences to help us realize that we are the *Purusha*. We become purified and refined, and our understanding expands. We cease to identify with the changing body and mind and recognize ourselves to be the unchanging Seer within.

The *Yoga Sutras of Patanjali* provides a roadmap to this awakening. A beautiful journey unfolds as one progresses from *sutra* to *sutra*. Given Patanjali's precision and clarity, however, there seems to be a glaring gap early in the exposition. In Book 1, *sutras 2–3*, the goal of Yoga is given as follows: "The restraint of the modifications of the mind-stuff is Yoga. Then the Seer [Self] abides in its own nature." Then, Book 1, *sutra* 4 states: "At other times, [the Self appears to] assume the forms of the mental modifications." Upon reflection, this false identification seems very strange. If the supreme power and intelligence of the universe dwells within us, as our own true nature, how would this error happen? There is obviously something missing here: a crucial clue to unraveling the mystery of the mind.

In Book 2, the mystery is solved: The mechanism of delusion is revealed as the *kleshas*, the five foundational obstacles, are introduced—ignorance, egoism, attachment, aversion, and clinging to bodily life. Ignorance is the field for all the rest, the seed from which the others sprout. It is defined as "regarding the impermanent as permanent, the impure as pure, the painful as pleasant, and the non-Self as the Self." The definition of egoism is then given as "the identification, as it were, of the power of the Seer with that of the instrument of seeing [body-mind]." Simply put, we forget who we are in truth and then we think we are something else. Therein lies the root of our delusion.

So, we come with this built-in design feature, the *kleshas*, and then the challenge becomes to find a way to bypass it—a way of knowing that transcends the limitations of the mind. The main technique toward this end in Raja Yoga is that of meditation. By focusing on one thing, our chosen object of meditation, the mind stops thinking many things. It becomes one-pointed, and when that focus is sustained, even that object slips away and the mind becomes still. In that stillness, we go beyond the mind, see to the depths of our being, and experience our true nature—the peace and bliss of the Self.

Bhakti Yoga

The path of Bhakti Yoga is also dualistic, but in a different way. Raja Yogis believe that *Purusha* and *Prakriti* are forever dualistic categories of existence. Bhakti Yogis begin by worshiping the Divine in a dualistic fashion, but, ultimately, they come to another understanding. Sri Ramakrishna Paramahamsa, a revered saint from India, described three levels of devotees. The first level sees God as different from the creation. The middle level understands God to be the inner guide that dwells within everyone's heart. But the highest level recognizes that God alone has become everything.

Depending on the particular sect, or faith tradition, there are various stories and legends to explain how God created the world—how the One (the eternal principle) became many (the ever-changing creation). In the book of Genesis in the *Holy Bible*, for example, first there is only God, and then God decides to create the universe. One can conclude that if there was only God, then the material out of which the universe was created must have been God. Swami Satchidananda explained the creation thus: God became bored being all alone and so created the universe, and then all the fun began. This creative activity is called *lila*, the play of the Divine. In the Hindu tradition, there is a well-known deity called Shiva Nataraja that depicts the five functions of the Divine: creation, preservation, destruction, veiling, and grace. This shows that both illusion and liberation are intrinsic features of the divine plan.

Whereas the Raja Yogi relies primarily on self-discipline to attain mastery over the mind, the Bhakti Yogi employs a more heart-centered approach. Bhakti Yoga practices include prayer, worship, chanting the names of God, and service to one and all as God in manifestation. The Bhakti Yogi transmutes emotion into pure devotion by cultivating a particular relationship with the Divine.

Traditionally, there are five *bhavas*, or attitudes, that characterize the different relationships one can have with God. In *shanta bhava*, the devotee rests peacefully in God. Sri Gurudev exemplified this approach when he used to say, "Peace is my God." In *dasya bhava*, the devotee is the servant of God. Hanuman, the servant of Lord Rama, exemplified this approach. Rama's wife, Sita, was kidnapped from India and taken to Sri Lanka. To rescue her, Rama had to build a bridge. But Hanuman, his great devotee, chanted Rama's name and leapt across the water.

Sakhya bhava is for those who regard God as a beloved friend. Arjuna had this relationship with Lord Krishna. During a war that occurred in ancient times, Krishna served as Arjuna's charioteer. On the battlefield, itself, Krishna imparted the teachings of the *Bhagavad Gita* to his beloved friend, Arjuna, to encourage and instruct him, so he would have proper understanding and perform his duty well. The *Holy Bible* praises the greatness of love between friends in this verse: "Greater love has no one than this, to lay down one's life for one's friends."

Vatsalya bhava is for those who worship God as their child. A pious devotee of Sri Ramakrishna named Gopaler Ma had this relationship with the baby Krishna, whose presence she experienced in divine, ecstatic visions. In *madhurya bhava*, one has the attitude of lover to the beloved. Both the Hindu saint, Mirabai, who lived in the 16th century, as well as the Sufi saint, Rabi'a al-'Adawiyya who lived in the 8th century, saw God in this light and composed beautiful, prayerful poems expressing their love.

We begin by conceiving of God in a limited way according to our taste, temperament, faith, and capacity. The Absolute God is nameless and formless, but it comes down to our level and manifests as countless forms in order to communicate with us. In Hinduism alone, there are thousands of names for God: like Shiva, Krishna, Muruga, Ganesh, Durga, Lakshmi, or Sarasvati. Since everything is an expression of God, we can approach the Divine through any name or form we choose. Eventually, we experience union with our beloved form of the Divine. Then, by the grace of the Divine, we are lifted even higher, beyond form, and we have the supreme realization.

For Sri Ramakrishna, this journey unfolded in an interesting way. He was an ardent devotee of the Goddess Kali and loved her so much he wasn't interested in experiencing the nameless, formless Absolute. He used to say, "The devotee of God wants to eat sugar, and not become sugar." One day, a wandering monk, by the name of Totapuri, who had experienced oneness with the Absolute, offered to guide him to that highest realization. Under Totapuri's direction, Sri Ramakrishna entered into meditation. When the Goddess appeared before him again, he used his discrimination as a sword and cut her form in two. His consciousness transcended beyond the realm of name and form, and he remained absorbed in *samadhi* for three days.

Jnana Yoga

Whereas the path for a Bhakti Yogi begins with a dualistic approach, the ultimate realization is of oneness. Jnana Yoga, on the other hand, employs a non-dualistic approach from the outset. The never-changing reality is termed as *Brahman*. It is all-pervasive, absolute consciousness, the eternal Witness. The world of diverse names and forms that we perceive constitutes the ever-changing. Although *Brahman* is unchanging and eternal, it appears as the changing world due to the actions of a mysterious, illusory power called *maya*. *Maya* is the agency of delusion. It conceals reality by superimposing the world on *Brahman*. Sri Swami Sivananda says, "It is difficult to conceive how the Infinite comes out of itself and becomes the finite. The magician can bring forth a rabbit out of a hat. We see it happening, but we cannot explain it; so, we call it *maya*, or illusion. *Maya* is a strange phenomenon, which cannot be accounted for by any law of nature. It is incapable of being described."

Adi Shankaracharya, a great proponent of non-dualism (or *Advaita)*, explained that the world is relatively real, while *Brahman* is absolutely real. The world appears real to one who is enveloped in ignorance due to *maya's* veil. But when knowledge of *Brahman* dawns and one experiences the unchanging reality, the illusory nature of the world becomes apparent. Compared to gazing at the ocean and seeing myriad fluctuations in the form of waves, bubbles, and foam—one now realizes that it's all just water temporarily assuming other forms.

There are five aspects to everything in creation: *sat, chid, ananda, nama,* and *rupa*, which translate as: existence, knowledge, bliss, name, and form. Existence-knowledge-bliss describes the essential nature; name and form refer to the changing manifestation. Normally, we only see the names and forms; when we realize *Brahman*, we perceive the underlying reality.

The practice of Jnana Yoga is a direct means to experiencing the truth of *Advaita*. This requires a keen intellect. Traditionally, a rigorous preparation was recommended. This included what were referred to as *Sadhana Chatushtaya*, the four means of salvation. They are: discrimination, dispassion, the six-fold qualities of perfection, and intense longing for liberation. The six-fold qualities are: serenity of mind, sense control, withdrawing from desire for sense enjoyment, endurance, faith, and concentration.

Unlike Raja Yoga, where you try to still the waves of the mind, Jnana Yoga techniques involve diving deep beneath the waves, where it is always peaceful. There are two levels to the mind: one part undergoes all the experiences, and the other part just watches. For example, if one day you inherit a lot of money, the mind will probably get excited. If the next day, someone steals the money, the mind may get depressed. But the awareness does not change: You know you are excited, and you know you are depressed.

Normally, we identify with the part of the mind that goes through all the changes. Our objective is to shift so that we identify with the level that is just watching. This will lead us, ultimately, to go beyond the mental level and experience the true Witness within. Then, the veil of *maya* will disappear, and we will have direct knowledge of the truth of Shankara's formula: *Brahma Satyam. Jagan Mithya. Jivo Brahmaiva Na'parah*, which means: "*Brahman* alone is real. The world is illusory. The individual is none other than *Brahman*."

Another technique is called *neti-neti* in which the aspirant consciously rejects as unreal everything that is subject to change. There's a story from olden times that illustrates how this works. There was a master sculptor who produced remarkable statues of elephants. After seeing one, the king decided to pay him a visit. He asked the sculptor if there was a secret behind his remarkable craftsmanship. The sculptor replied, "I go to the quarry, select a piece of marble, and bring it back to my studio. Then, I just remove all that is not elephant, and what remains is elephant." After rejecting everything that is imperfect, impure, and impermanent, we eventually realize that which is the eternal epitome of perfection and purity—the all-pervading supreme consciousness. The application of this technique requires constant remembrance and heightened awareness.

Years ago, at the San Francisco Integral Yoga Institute, a friend once brought us a large bag of walnuts that he had just harvested from his tree. So, we decided to have walnuts for dessert after lunch. We each got the same amount of walnuts and a nutcracker. After a while, I became aware that the fellow next to me had a totally different approach to eating walnuts. He was cracking them one at a time, and then immediately eating the nut. I, on the other hand, was cracking them and eliminating all that was not walnut, amassing a pile of nuts that I ate only at the end. Clearly, he was delighting in the sweetness of the walnut experience throughout the process. My path involved delayed fulfillment, but in the end, I enjoyed all the sweetness as well. He was a *bhakta* and I, a *jnani*, when it came to eating walnuts. We had our preferred methods, but in the end, we both were in walnut bliss.

As each of us is a blend of will, emotion, and intellect, we may employ elements of the various approaches at different times. On my own path, I have observed that when faced with mild challenges, I use my will and focus my mind to overcome them. For bigger challenges, I generally step back, observe, and analyze. But for really difficult situations, I go deep within my heart and seek the grace and guidance of the Divine. Whatever strategy we take, our aim is to maintain our peace and balance as we move through life and, ultimately, to wake up—to transcend the ever-changing and experience the never-changing bliss of our own true nature.

Exit Strategy for Suffering

Everyone wants to be happy, but the happiness we seek is elusive. Our lives are spent seeking happiness through possessions, positions, relationships; even our addictions are a misguided search for happiness. And what do we find? Generally, we get a little happiness mixed with a lot of problems and pain.

A little analysis will show that, if we expect permanent happiness through external attainments, we are destined for frustration and failure. This is because everything external is part of nature and, as such, is subject to change. Think of all that has changed in your own life over the past ten years: all the people who have come and gone, changes in your living situation, your work, your finances, your health, or simply how you spend your days. In everyone's life, the pendulum swings between pleasure and pain, loss and gain, praise and blame.

In the midst of all the change, where is the happiness that we are seeking? Raja Yoga provides an answer: Our essential nature is that supreme happiness. It's as if we are looking for our glasses, while all the time they are perched on top of our head.

Our true nature is happiness. As Swami Satchidananda often said, to experience one's true nature is like trying to see your own face. To see your face, you need a mirror. We have a mirror within—the mind. If the mirror of the mind is straight and clean, we see an accurate reflection and experience the peace and joy within. However, if the mirror is colored, curved, or twisted, we see a distorted reflection. Even though we are still perfectly fine, we see that reflection and think that's who we are. Because of this false identification, we suffer in life.

We forget our true nature, and then we look for external things to make us feel better, which only perpetuates the problem. First of all, as was already stated, we can never find lasting happiness this way because everything external is subject to constant change. And secondly, every time the mind goes outward to experience objects, it takes their form and gets colored by them. Thus, the mental mirror is continually distorting, and we never get to see the true reflection.

The very act of seeking happiness outside prevents us from experiencing the true happiness within. Instead, if we restrained the mind from going outward and let it rest calmly within, we would experience the happiness we are seeking. This is the essential teaching of Raja Yoga. When we forget our true nature and seek happiness outside ourselves, that is the basic ignorance, and the root of all suffering.

This situation leads us to some ultimate questions: Why don't we remember our true nature? Why do we identify with the distorted reflection? Why is there suffering? An explanation is provided in the *Yoga Sutras of Patanjali*, in which the teachings of Raja Yoga are presented. Raja Yoga can be understood as an exploration into the nature of suffering and how to overcome it. Patanjali speaks of basic defects, or afflictions, of the mind called *kleshas*. These are the underlying cause of suffering.

Ignorance (*avidya*) is the first *klesha*. It's defined as regarding the impermanent as permanent, the impure as pure, the painful as pleasant, and the non-Self as the Self. We don't understand who we are. We forget our true nature and, if that weren't bad enough, we think we are something else. That's when the next *klesha*, egoism (*asmita*), comes in. We identify with what is closest to us, the mind and the body, and we think that's who we are.

Then we become attached to all that we find pleasurable and averse to all that is painful. This is known as *raga* and *dvesha*. We are ever running toward things we think will make us happy and away from things we find painful, leaving little time for simply staying still, poised, balanced, resting in the supreme happiness within. The final *klesha* is clinging to bodily life (*abhinivesha*). We cling to the body because we think that defines our existence, who we are. Additionally, we have had many births and died many times before, leaving painful *samskaras* (mental impressions) associated with death in the deeper levels of the mind.

You can picture the *kleshas* as a clever design feature, integrated into the fundamental hardwiring of the mental computer. We are hardwired to approach life and to see things in a distorted way. Our sense organs can only function within a limited range. We can't even hear sounds, for example, that are audible to a dog or a bat. Imagine how different the world would look if we had microscopic eyes. As a vegetarian, we couldn't even comfortably drink a glass of water! Then, this input gets interpreted by a mind that is also running interpretive software based on all the conditioning it has received from family, friends, society, schooling, religion, etc. We are trying to understand the truth, using a limited instrument that is incapable of totally grasping it and distorts what it can grasp.

We are steeped in ignorance. We forget the peace and joy that is our true nature, and we seek happiness outside ourselves. The world is just not set up to give us lasting happiness. In fact, its purpose is to teach us the contrary, that one has to go beyond the limitations of the body, senses, and mind to experience true joy.

Patanjali recognized this predicament when he said that to one of discrimination, everything is painful. We invest so much effort to get what we want. Once we get it, however, there are three problematic consequences: (1) There may be anxiety or fear over losing what has been gained. (2) The resultant impressions left in the mind from the pleasure of attaining a desired object will give rise to new cravings. In other words, fulfilling a desire only fans the flame; it's like pouring oil on fire. (3) The mind is never satisfied for long. The mind, itself, is part of nature, and as such, is subject to constant change. So, what gave us pleasure on one day, no longer satisfies us the next.

So, how do we bypass this hardwiring, short-circuit this predicament, and find true happiness? How is it possible to cease to identify with the body and mind, and transcend suffering? The story that Sri Gurudev told of Sri Ramana Maharshi shows that it can be done. In his later years, Sri Ramana developed cancer on the arm. He just wanted to let the karma purge itself out. However, his disciples wanted to treat it and called a doctor.

The doctor came and announced that surgery was necessary, so Sri Ramana consented. However, when the surgeon went to administer anesthesia, Sri Ramana refused. The doctor cautioned him, saying that it was going to be a very painful procedure, but Sri Ramana just told him to proceed.

The doctor performed the surgery, and as others watched, so did Sri Ramana. In fact, he spoke to his arm in the following manner: "You must have gotten into a lot of mischief before, because look at all the suffering you are having to endure. Well, face it and purge it out." How could he do this so calmly? He could do so because he wasn't identified with the body or the mind. He was established in his true Self. The *Bhagavad Gita* describes Yoga as, "disconnecting your identification with that which experiences pain," in other words, the body and mind. Sri Ramana was established in that state of realization, and we can attain it as well.

Through the teachings of Raja Yoga, we are presented with a skillful way to accomplish this goal. A simple analogy will help us to understand the underlying method. Imagine, for a moment, how an automobile runs. The movement of the piston gets transferred to the wheels, and then the car moves. When we wish to stop the car, we don't apply the brakes to the piston where the movement began. Instead, we apply them to the wheels, the most visible expression of the movement, and then everything gets stopped in the reverse order.

Going back to the *kleshas*, we want to dispel ignorance, which is the beginning of the chain that results in all suffering in life. So, we begin by addressing the most visible expression of ignorance, which is attachment. *Raga, dvesha,* and *abhinivesha* are all expressions of attachment. We are attached to the body, to all that gives us pleasure, and to avoiding all that causes us pain. If we can let go of our attachments, our minds will become peaceful, and we will be able to experience our true nature.

The essential question, then, is how do we let go of attachment? Patanjali gives us the method in Book 1, *sutra* 12, which states, "The mind is brought under control by practice and non-attachment." It's very difficult to let go of our desires and attachments; that's why a two-sided approach is needed. Through practice we gain the strength and clarity to release our attachments.

Sri Gurudev would often say that the practices are like soaps. Hatha Yoga is soap for the physical body; *pranayama* is soap for the subtle body; and meditation is soap for the mind. Rather than tell someone to stop doing a harmful behavior, he would tell that person to just practice Yoga. If someone wished to stop smoking, for example, he would recommend *bhastrika pranayama* to clear out the nicotine deposits in the lungs. Once the lungs were clear, the craving would cease, and the smoking habit would just fall away.

Yoga never speaks of suppression. If you suppress a desire, it will only spring back forcefully when you relax your vigilance or are a little weak. Instead, it says to attach and detach. Just start doing the positive, and automatically you'll stop doing the negative. Engage in Yoga practice and, eventually, you will be able to resolve and release your attachments. When the mind is free of all desire and attachment, it becomes pure and steady, and we experience our true Self. This approach constitutes the underlying methodology that is threaded throughout the *Yoga Sutras*. It is, in effect, Patanjali's main exit strategy for overcoming suffering.

Prescriptions for Peace

Our whole experience of life is based on the stories we tell ourselves about what occurs. These stories begin with our mind's interpretation of what it perceives. Swami Vivekananda describes this like an oyster making a pearl. A parasite gets inside the shell, and then the oyster reacts to the irritation by producing enamel around it, which is then called a pearl. Actual events that occur are like the parasite; all that we ever know are the pearls created by our own minds. We are not able to perceive the raw incoming data because, immediately, our minds react to it. In the *Yoga Sutras of Patanjali*, these reactions or activities of the mind are described as *vrittis*. Our known universe consists of these *vrittis*, the thought-waves of the mind.

Like the ebb and flow of the ocean, with waves breaking upon the shore, the world as we know it is, thus, subject to constant change. The goal of Yoga is to calm the waves of the mind so we can see to its depths and experience the ground of our being—the peace, balance, and stability of our own true nature. Then we will experience true happiness and freedom.

The Thought-waves

In the *Yoga Sutras*, Patanjali presents the philosophy of Yoga, and shows himself to be, not only a master of the yogic science, but also a skillful teacher with great insight as to how to lead students, step by step to the goal. In Book 1, first he tells us that, in order to attain the goal of Yoga, we need to totally control the *vrittis*, the thought-waves of the mind. Immediately after, he describes the *vrittis*, telling us that there are five kinds. When you consider how many millions of thoughts we have in a given day, the prospect of bringing them all under control must have seemed quite daunting to his students. But, if there are only five kinds, then the task becomes doable. Instead of being overwhelmed and discouraged, we feel empowered and motivated. The five kinds of *vrittis* are: right knowledge, misconception, verbal delusion (sometimes referred to as imagination or conceptualization), sleep, and memory. They are either painful or painless, depending on whether our intention is selfish or selfless.

The Obstacles

In Book 2, Patanjali examines the underlying dynamic that causes the *vrittis*. These are the *kleshas*, the fundamental obstacles, or basic afflictions, of the mind. Primary among them and the field for all the others is ignorance of our true nature, or *avidya*. We forget our true nature, the divine Spirit within us that is ever peaceful and joyful. Then, we identify with what is closest to us, the mind and the body, and think that's who we are. This constitutes the next *klesha*, known as *asmita*, or egoism. This is problematic because, unlike our true nature, the mind and body are constantly changing. So instead of having a reliable lens with which to navigate through life, it's as if we have a kaleidoscopic one. We become attached to what we find pleasurable and averse to all that is painful *(raga and dvesha)*. We find ourselves continually buffeted by shifting currents, known as the dualities in life. In the midst of all the ups and downs, we cling to bodily life because we think that defines our existence and because memories of the pain of death remain in the subconscious mind from prior births. This is the final *klesha (abhinivesha)*.

The *kleshas* are the root cause of "dis-ease" in life. When there is an underlying ailment, there are usually observable symptoms. Likewise, the *kleshas* give rise to certain "symptoms" in life. These are presented in Book 1 as the common obstacles encountered on the spiritual path. They are described as *chittavikshepa*, distractions of the mind-stuff. There are nine obstacles: disease, dullness, doubt, carelessness, laziness, sensuality, false perception, failure to reach firm ground, and slipping from the ground gained. Accompaniments to the obstacles include: distress, despair, trembling of the body, and disturbed breathing. So there are two levels of obstacles presented in the *Yoga Sutras:* the fundamental ones that are more permanent, and the more superficial ones that may or may not be in play at any given time.

Like an expert physician, Patanjali first looks at the symptoms in Book 1. Then, in Book 2, he goes deeper and identifies the underlying cause. After assessing the situation, in Book 2, *sutra 16*, he boldly proclaims that the situation is curable, "Pain that has not yet come is avoidable." It is one of the most life-affirming, hope-filled statements in the entire text. If this sounds like a medical analysis, according to tradition, Patanjali is believed to have authored not only the *Yoga Sutras,* but a medical text as well.

The Meditation Pathway

Just like a good physician recognizes that people with the same illness may require different courses of treatment and prescriptions due to their particular constitution and preferences, Patanjali provides alternative pathways for aspirants seeking spiritual realization. The first pathway is gaining mastery over the mind by directly controlling the thoughts. This is the path of meditation. In Book 1, *sutra* 2, he gives the goal of Yoga: "The restraint of the modifications of the mind-stuff is Yoga." Then, in Book 1, *sutra* 12, he tells us how to accomplish this restraint: "These mental modifications are restrained by practice and non-attachment." Both practice and non-attachment are needed to go deep in meditation. Practice is defined as "effort toward steadiness of mind." In order to steady the mind, you train it to focus on one point, your chosen object of meditation. Non-attachment is about freedom from craving, letting go of desires that dissipate, distract, or disturb the mind. If you practice without non-attachment, it is like trying to move in opposite directions at the same time; you won't make it to your goal.

Imagine if you develop an allergic rash. Seeking relief, you go to the doctor. The doctor will likely take a two-sided approach. First, the doctor will prescribe an ointment to calm the rash. But that is not enough: it's also essential to determine what is causing the problem and stay away from that. Otherwise, you might apply a lot of ointment (like doing practice), but you won't eliminate the rash unless you also stop exposing yourself to the irritant (non-attachment).

The Devotional Pathway

Shortly after exploring this approach, Patanjali offers another pathway for attaining the goal. In Book 1, *sutra* 23, he announces: "Or [*samadhi* is attained] by devotion with total dedication to God." This seminal *sutra,* which seems to suddenly appear, is all the more remarkable when one considers that this is a radical departure from the *Sankhya* metaphysics upon which the *Yoga Sutras* is based; *Sankhya* contains no such concept of God. It almost feels like Patanjali is giving us a chance to attain the goal in an easier way, if we have the faith and temperament to do so.

How can we understand the equivalent effectiveness of these two approaches? Our goal is to make the mind calm and clean. When it is calm and clean, it is like a pure lake. We can see to the depths of our being and experience our true Self. We can attain this stillness through meditation, in which we directly cultivate one thought, our object of meditation. When we become perfectly one-pointed, even that thought slips away, and we rest in the peace of our true nature.

We can also attain this state if we totally surrender and accept the divine will in all things, because, then the mind will retain its peace no matter what happens. If we love God with our entire mind, we will have found an indirect method to control our thoughts. The following story illustrates this point.

An actor once met Sri Ramakrishna and asked to be his disciple. After professing his love for the saint, the actor added that he was addicted to cigarettes and alcohol. He also confessed to frequenting houses of prostitution and did not wish to relinquish any of his bad habits. Sri Ramakrishna accepted him as his disciple with one qualification: Every time he was about to engage in one of those habits, he would have to offer it first to him.

The actor departed happy, having gotten his wish. That night, after a performance, he sat down and lit up a cigarette. He raised it to his lips and pronounced: "In the name of Sri Ramakrishna." He immediately stopped short, thinking to himself, "How can I smoke in his name? He would never do such a thing." So, he put it out. He proceeded to pour himself a glass of whiskey, and the same thing ensued. He went to a brothel and found himself in a similar predicament. Because he truly loved his Guru and saw the divine in him, he could no longer do those things in his Guru's name. In this manner, the actor's weaknesses were readily overcome.

Integrating Both Approaches

Patanjali presents us with alternative pathways to reach our destination: a devotional solution, as well as the meditative approach. In offering these two pathways, perhaps he was subtly suggesting that they be integrated. Even in his discussion of the two levels of obstacles in Books 1 and 2, he frames them between *sutras* that describe ways to overcome them through devotion or meditation, underscoring the importance of both methods.

There are common elements in both pathways. For example, prayer and worship are forms of meditation. Following the devotional path—living in accordance with God's will and offering everything to the Divine—entails effort (practice) and lifestyle adjustments (non-attachment). Total surrender doesn't come that easily either. For most seekers, some effort is involved in maintaining that perspective in life. Swami Satchidananda used to speak of kitten and monkey devotion. The kitten just cries, and the mother cat grasps it by the scruff of the neck and carries it along. The monkey, however, clings to the belly of the mother as she jumps from tree to tree. Both rely on the mother, but the monkey exerts effort as well.

And if we pursue the path of meditation relying solely on self-effort, there's the risk that along with our spiritual progress, our ego may inflate as well. Sri Gurudev even says, "Ultimately, nobody can achieve eternal peace by doing something with the mind, which is part of nature. That supreme joy can only be acquired when you rise above nature by complete surrender." In other words, self-effort alone can only take us so far when the mind is trying to control the mind, in order to transcend the mind. But self-effort—along with the humility, receptivity, and gratitude that come from a devotional perspective—will ensure our success.

With the spirit of devotion, the journey will be sweet. With the focus of meditation, it will be efficient. Together, they're a perfect prescription for overcoming all obstacles and attaining the highest.

One Practice Is All You Need

In the *Yoga Sutras*, Sri Patanjali Maharishi lists nine obstacles, which cover a range of physical, mental, and spiritual problems. They are: disease, dullness, doubt, carelessness, laziness, sensuality, false perception, failure to reach firm ground, and slipping from the ground gained. He states that they are accompanied by distress, despair, trembling of the body, and disturbed breathing. He is a very gentle and skillful teacher, so immediately before presenting this formidable and all-too-familiar list, he reassures us that a single practice can make all these obstacles disappear. This potent panacea is mantra *japa*.

Why is mantra *japa* so effective? To understand this, it's helpful to explore a little cosmology, the science that explains the origins of the universe. The ancient yogis noted that the universe oscillates through cycles of potentiality and manifestation. When a new cycle is to begin, the first expression is sound. If you think of the physical universe as a grand machine, then this could be understood as the hum of an engine as it starts up. The yogis refer to this primordial sound as the *pranava*, the cosmic hum. The *Holy Bible* declares: "In the beginning was the Word, and the Word was with God, and the Word was God." The ancient Hindu scripture, the *Rig Veda*, echoes the same truth: "In the beginning was *Brahman*, with whom was the Word, and the Word was truly the supreme *Brahman*."

As creation proceeded, variations of the original hum began to vibrate on different levels, giving rise to all the multifarious forms. So the entire creation—everyone and everything—is nothing but sound vibrations in different wavelengths. Each one of us has our own unique vibratory signature, which results from all the physical and mental, gross and subtle, activity that is occurring within us.

Even scientists tell us that musical production can be found everywhere in nature. The whole cosmos is like a grand symphony, in which our planet earth lends its own particular hum. Several years back, astronomers detected the deepest note ever observed in the cosmos, a

B-flat that is fifty-seven octaves below middle C. They say it has been sounding through space for about two-and-a-half billion years.

Now, if you think of God as a cosmic radio transmitter, mantras represent particular divine frequencies that are being broadcast. We are all like radio receiving sets. If we tune in, we get the music. We experience the Divine, because we are vibrating at that level. All knowledge and power flow through us. On the other hand, if we're not properly tuned, we may get a lot of static, resulting in confusion and delusion.

Japa, the repetition of a mantra, enables us to do that tuning. Mantras are mystic sound structures that were revealed to sages in deep meditation. They are divine power expressing through sound. Through the concentrated repetition of a mantra over time, we begin to vibrate in a new way, at a higher divine frequency.

Just like we use sound vibrations to clean items like jewels, teeth, or even kidney stones, mantras clean our entire system—physical and mental. Swami Sivananda, who was a physician before becoming a monk, states: "Chronic diseases can be cured by mantras. The chanting of mantras generates potent spiritual waves and divine vibrations. The mantra vibrations penetrate the physical and astral bodies of the patients and remove the cause of their suffering. They fill the cells with pure *sattva* and divine energy. They destroy microbes and rejuvenate the cells and tissues." If you think of disease as disharmonious vibrations in cells, tissues, and organs, then mantras can be understood as establishing pure, clean, harmonious vibrations. When everything is vibrating at this new level, health is restored.

Mantras clean, heal, and attune us to the Divine. They can also protect us from danger, which I experienced firsthand years ago at our Connecticut *ashram*. I was in the habit of taking long walks at dusk. There is a palpable presence of peace at that time. It's as if the earth, itself, exhales, releasing the tensions of the day, as it heads toward the deep relaxation of night.

Once when I was on such a walk, enjoying the quiet solitude, I noticed on a nearby hillside a very large dog. I recognized him as one that had attacked several of the men at the *ashram*. Our eyes locked for a moment, and then the dog began charging down the hill in my direction.

It was a deserted area; there was no one in sight. At moments like this, one remembers to pray. So, I clasped my hands, gazed up, and uttered, "God, if it's Your will for me to be torn to shreds by a wild dog, an opportunity is fast approaching." Then, I proceeded to repeat my mantra. Within seconds, the dog was before me, repeatedly rushing at me, but somehow, never touching me. He kept opening and closing his jaws around my fingers, but never made contact. I slowly kept walking, and eventually the dog ran off.

I continued my walk for another half-mile and then had to return. The only way back was the way I had come, and once again, I found myself opposite the hillside where the dog was waiting. I folded my hands, uttered the same prayer, and repeated the mantra. Again, our eyes locked, and he came storming my way. The same bizarre dance ensued in which he repeatedly charged and went to bite, but never made contact. Finally, he ran off, and I returned to the *ashram*.

The next day at work we were playing a tape of Swami Satchidananda in which he was speaking about the power of the mantra. He said if you develop the vibration through repetition, it will form a protective shield around you. In Sanskrit, this is called *kavacham*, which means armor. He said you could even be in the jungle, and animals might come to attack, but they will never touch you. An invisible mantric shield will protect you from all harm.

You can select a mantra yourself, or request one from your teacher, if you have found your spiritual path. The ceremony in which you receive a mantra is called initiation. At that time, the teacher not only imparts the mantra, but also transmits a little spiritual energy to enliven it within you.

If we make the mantra a constant companion, it will be the greatest friend, a steady anchor at all times. It can heal the body, lift the spirit, open the heart, and expand the mind. A mantra is like soap; it cleanses the body and mind. It is like fire; it burns all the impurities. Repetition of the mantra will make the mind strong, clear, and collected.

As our practice deepens, our minds will become more absorbed in the mantra. Instead of many thoughts, we become established in that one pure thought. At that point, when the mind is really strong, the mantra will dissolve, and the mind will be still. In that stillness, the true Self is revealed. In that state, we realize that we are not the body, not the mind, but the immortal Spirit. With that knowledge, all obstacles disappear. We have attained liberation, freedom from suffering, and will experience supreme peace and bliss.

Freedom through Meditation

Spiritual life is all about freedom. How free are you?

I made an unexpected discovery in this regard early in my spiritual journey, when I was living in Philadelphia. One night, I was comfortably lying in bed beginning to drift off to sleep, when all of a sudden, I heard a whisper within my mind—one word: "Pizza." I rolled over and tried to get back to sleep. Within a few moments, louder this time, I heard it again: "Pizza, pizza, P-I-Z-Z-A!" No matter how much I tried to ignore it, it kept reasserting itself, until it seemed like a "pizza parade" was marching through my consciousness. Like an unwilling bystander, I watched as this rogue desire got me out of bed, dressed, and on the way to an all-night shop to have some pizza. Clearly, this was not freedom. Freedom entails the capacity to choose, to evaluate a situation and make a good decision. In this case, to be able to say to the mind, "No, this is not a good idea now. If you still want pizza tomorrow, you can have it for lunch."

Most of us, most of the time, are not aware of how enslaved we are. We are like unwitting puppets, animated by the strings of desires, memories, habits, and emotions that inhabit the deeper levels of the mind. Through spiritual practice, we can come to release this bondage, so we can experience more freedom as we move through life, and, ultimately, be free of all limitations.

This is where meditation is especially effective. Meditation is the science of gaining mastery over the mind. Our whole experience of life is based on the condition of the mind—how we perceive and respond to situations. We don't see things as they are, but through a mental filter that is colored by our prior conditioning. It's like each one of us is wearing a particular type of glasses. The lenses could be rosy, green convex, yellow concave, purple prismatic, or any other variation. Through meditation, we come to recognize the glasses we are wearing and gain the capacity to remove them. Only then can we see clearly and realize the higher truth. And as the *Holy Bible* states, "The truth shall set you free."

The end of meditation is freedom, and so is the beginning. Based on our taste, temperament, capacity, and faith, we can select any method that works for us.

There are four basic approaches to meditation: focusing on an object, witnessing, Self-inquiry, and prayer. They all involve shifting into a mode of greater awareness through applied attention, but the techniques vary as follows.

Focusing on an Object

To understand the focusing approach, picture the mind like a lake. At the bottom of the lake is a priceless jewel, the true Self, which is perfect peace and joy. Every thought, feeling, perception, or memory colors and causes a wave in the mental lake, so that we can't see clearly to the depths of our being. If we can restrain the mind from forming into waves and make it calm and clean, there will be no distortion, and we will be able to experience our true Self. It is very difficult to go from many waves to no waves, so the technique involves setting up one pure, powerful wave—the object of our meditation. We restrain the mind from many things by focusing on one thing. We consciously cultivate one thought-form in the mind, and when that becomes steady, it, too, slips away. So, we go from many to one, and then from one to none and, in that stillness, we experience the peace of our true nature.

The object of our focus can be a sound, a form, or an idea. In the *Yoga Sutras of Patanjali,* we are given the freedom to choose anything we like that is elevating. The object is important because as the mind becomes more absorbed in the object, we imbibe those qualities. The first stage of practice is called *dharana,* or concentration. At that stage, we are trying to fix the mind on our object, but it repeatedly wanders, and we bring it back. The second stage is called *dhyana,* or meditation. At this point, the mind has become more settled, and there is a continuous flow of cognition toward the object. In the final stage, known as *samadhi,* there is the super-conscious experience when the mind becomes totally absorbed in its object.

An everyday comparison can help make this clear. *Dharana* is like dating—the mind is playing the field. *Dhyana* is when you've made a commitment to one partner, and you devote all your attention to your chosen one. And *samadhi* can be compared to the experience of bliss when you unite with your beloved. The Chinese poet, Li Po, beautifully described the experience of absorption:

> The birds have vanished in the sky,
> and now the last cloud drains away.
> We sit together, the mountain and I
> until only the mountain remains.

Witnessing

The mind functions on different levels. One part of the mind goes through all the fluctuations, but another part is always watching. This principle is employed in the witnessing approach to meditation. Imagine that you are in a movie theater watching a film in which you are also playing a starring role. So you are in the audience, as well as on the screen. If you can identify with the Witness in the audience, rather than with the character on the screen, you will keep your peace no matter what unfolds. Likewise, instead of identifying with the part of the mind that is going through all the ups and downs, you can learn to identify with the stable part of the mind that is simply aware of all that is happening. In Sanskrit, this is called *sakshitvam bhavana*, the witnessing attitude.

The technique involves simply observing the thoughts as they come and go, like clouds passing before the sun. Rather than trying to control the thoughts, you detach from them. When you detach from mental activity, it's like turning off a main switch. The mind will slow down. It's our identification with the thoughts that energizes them. Consider the mind like a mischievous child. If nobody is watching, the child will do whatever it wants. But if a child knows the mother is watching, it will behave properly. In the same way, if you watch the mind, it will calm down and stop all its pranks. Confucius said, "It's better to light one small candle than to curse the darkness." Instead of struggling with the thoughts, the light of awareness dispels them.

Begin by identifying with the witnessing level of the mind. This level of the mind resembles the true Witness within, the pure consciousness of the Self. After continually cultivating this awareness over time, with one part of the mind watching the other, you will eventually transcend the mental level altogether and experience the true Witness within.

Self-inquiry

There is another approach to meditation called Self-inquiry, which involves direct analysis. You can begin by posing the question: "Who am I?" and observe the responses that come. Usually, the answers will reflect identification with conditions or relationships based on the body or mind, such as: "I am a teenager," "I am a mother," "I am a carpenter," or "I am an American." As the body and mind are subject to change, question who you are without these identifications. If you keep negating all such answers, eventually, you will experience the "I am" without any qualifiers. You will realize your true Self.

Or you can begin by witnessing the mind and when thoughts arise, question the thoughts themselves: "Where did this thought come from? How did it come? Whose thought is this? How do I know this? Who am I then?" A little analysis will reveal that anything you can observe is not you. You are the subject and the shifting thoughts are the object of your awareness. This technique helps you to transcend the changing landscape of the mind and attunes you to the eternal Witness within.

I had a profound experience of this technique years ago when I was living at the San Francisco IYI. I was having one of those meditations where the mind was overflowing with non-stop chatter. Finally, at one point, I asked the question: "Who is doing all this talking?" Suddenly and unexpectedly, from a place deep within, a very clear, calm, and centered voice replied: "And who is listening?" Everything stopped, and there was utter silence, stillness, and peace.

Prayer

Prayer can also be a form of meditation. Compared to the other techniques, it is an indirect approach. You don't deal with the thoughts directly as in focusing, witnessing, or questioning. Instead, you redirect your attention to God and offer everything—all your thoughts, feelings, petitions, and praises—to God. You place everything in God's hands and accept whatever comes as God's will for your highest good. If you have that sort of faith and acceptance, the mind will retain its peace. In this way, the devotional approach can be a shortcut to enlightenment.

For prayer to be effective, it must be rooted in faith and accompanied by heartfelt feeling. Swami Satchidananda likens prayer to a connecting wire. God is the main battery, and we are like light bulbs. It is the intimate outpouring from the heart of the devotee to the Divine that establishes the connection. When our prayer is one-pointed, we make a good connection, and the Higher Power flows through us. We begin by focusing on the meaning of every word, but as our prayer deepens, the words fall away. We enter into the silence and experience the peace and presence of God.

Comparison and Combining of Techniques

In focusing, we control the thoughts by consciously developing one pure, powerful thought—the object of our meditation. In witnessing, we detach from the thoughts. In Self-inquiry, we analyze the thoughts. And in prayer, we offer the thoughts to God.

Prayer and witnessing are similar in that they align us at the outset with the higher consciousness, except the first is devotional and dualistic, whereas the second is intellectual and monistic. Eventually, prayer leads to the monistic state when the devotee experiences union with the Divine. The great philosopher Adi Shankaracharya proclaimed that *parabhakti* (supreme devotion) and *parajnanam* (supreme wisdom) ultimately bring us to the same realization. So, even though the path is very different for the one who pursues prayer and the one who prefers witnessing, the final destination is the same. A living example of this confluence of devotion and wisdom, Shankara expounded the highest *Vedanta*, a non-dualistic, intellectual approach, as well as saw himself as a child of the Divine Mother and composed soul-stirring devotional poetry.

In our personal practice, we can even have our own unique blend of these techniques. For example, no matter which method we use, we can begin and end our sitting with prayer. Initially, we can ask for guidance and invoke blessings. At the end, we can express our gratitude and offer our meditation for the well-being of all creation.

If you focus on a mantra as your main practice, you can employ witnessing before the mantra repetition. To do this, after your opening routine, just sit still and watch the mind. When it looks for something to do, then begin repeating the mantra. You could repeat the mantra as a prayer, or you could continue in a witnessing mode, watching or listening to the repetition. If your central practice is prayer, you can combine it with focusing on an image of your beloved form of the Divine. Once you've selected your method, stick with it and go deep.

Whatever approach we choose, we gain greater clarity, strength, balance, and perspective. More and more in our daily lives, the dimension of choice begins to enter. We are able to see more options and have a growing capacity to respond rather than react to situations. Ultimately, we experience the highest consciousness. Then we are really free.

Breath: The Subtle Connection

Often in life, we overlook the value of the simple and familiar: a kind word, a helping hand, a timely smile. Such everyday gestures impart meaning and a sense of connectedness as we wend our way through time and space. Similarly, the breath is our constant companion, yet seldom do we realize the pivotal connecting role it plays in our existence and the great power and mystery that lie hidden in its effortless flow.

All life on the planet is connected through the breath. We dwell within a common atmosphere, which we continually draw into ourselves, process, and then give back to. We exchange molecules and partake of one another through this flow of energy. Perhaps some of the molecules that were within a butterfly a few moments ago, or were part of the Buddha over 2000 years ago, are now circulating as our own body or mind. The simple act of breathing renders us all intimately connected, and not separate, distinct entities. As Swami Satchidananda used to say, "We are cells of one universal body."

Breath is our very life. In the *Bible* we read that God formed Adam out of inert matter and breathed life into him. Approximately fifteen times per minute, or 21,600 times a day, the Higher Power continues to do so in each of us today. With each exhalation, we are on the brink of "expiration." If it didn't return, we'd die. Yet, without any forethought on our part, the Higher Power keeps sending it back as long as there's more for us to do.

When we inhale, along with the air, we take in *prana*, the vital energy that sustains all creation. While we can live for minutes without air, we wouldn't even survive a moment without *prana*. We also obtain *prana* from the sun, water, and food we consume. It is the life force that permeates and animates every particle of the universe. Wherever there is movement on any level—from the most outer, gross, physical movements to the most inner, subtle, mental ones—it is powered by *prana*.

The movement of the earth through the heavens, the wind blowing through the trees, the ebb and flow of the tides, the gasoline that powers a car, the electricity that charges a computer, the physiological processes that maintain the life of an organism—are all expressions of *prana*. Even the passage of thoughts through the mind is made possible by *prana*. It is *prana* that causes all the movements within an individual—both physical and mental. So, by controlling the *pranic* currents within, we can optimize our physical and mental well-being.

The goal of Yoga is to still the mind so we can experience the supreme peace and joy that is our true nature. This is the most challenging task, one that has been compared to trying to tame a drunken monkey that has been bitten by a scorpion. While it may be very difficult to directly control the mind, if we can regulate the energy that moves the thoughts, we will have found an indirect route for achieving our goal.

The control of the *prana* is accomplished through the yogic science of *pranayama*, which involves regulating the breath. We focus on the breath because it is a grosser, external manifestation of the *prana*. By controlling it, we gain control of the subtler *prana* within.

Additionally, among all our physiological processes, the breath is unique in that it can be either voluntary or involuntary. Our entry point is voluntary control, and this, in turn, gives us access to controlling the so-called involuntary functions within. Adept yogis have demonstrated that even the heartbeat and brainwaves can be altered, or even stopped, if one knows how to direct the *prana*.

When we learn how to control the *prana* within, we gain mastery over the cosmic *prana* as well. Our bodies are a microcosm of the universe. The same laws that govern the *prana* within our bodies pertain in the macrocosm as well. Picture a group of scientists who wish to learn about seawater. It would be impossible for them to bring the entire ocean into their laboratory. Instead, they analyze the water in a small beaker, with the understanding that the water in the ocean would be the same. Similarly, within the laboratory of our spiritual practice, our bodies are like little beakers of the cosmic *prana*. We learn about the cosmic force within ourselves, and it is the same force that is functioning on other levels throughout the universe.

There are three basic ways we can relate to the breath: Through *pranayama*, we regulate it. For pain management and *pranic* healing, we visualize and direct it. As a meditation practice, we observe it.

Regulating the Breath

The science of *pranayama* offers techniques that can energize, strengthen, detoxify, relax, and heat or cool the body. There are methods to calm, balance, fortify, focus, and uplift the mind. Through regular practice, the dormant spiritual energy within, known as *kundalini*, is awakened leading to an expanded state of awareness. All this is possible simply from working with the breath.

Sri Gurudev was once asked if it was better not to do *pranayama* in cities where there was a lot of pollution. He responded that even if the air was polluted, the *prana* always remains pure. And, he added, that is why we continue to be able to live in such challenging environments.

In speaking to a group dealing with HIV, the main practice Sri Gurudev recommended was to incorporate the basic three-part, deep, diaphragmatic breathing, known as *dirgha svasam*, throughout the day in order to rebuild the immune system. This simple technique, the foundation of all the other breathing practices, fills the lungs to capacity and empties them thoroughly, supercharging the system with oxygen and *prana*. The lymph system, which detoxifies the cells, is activated by deep breathing, so elimination of poisons and wastes is enhanced. The movement of the diaphragm also produces a gentle massaging action that improves the functioning of the heart and the various organs in the abdominal cavity.

For healing, in general, Gurudev recommended working up gradually to three, 30-minute *pranayama* sessions per day. Unless contraindicated by one's condition, a routine that involved three to five rounds of rapid diaphragmatic breathing (either *kapalabhati* or *bhastrika*), followed by five to ten minutes of alternate nostril breathing (either *nadi suddhi* or *sukha purvaka*), would be ideal. Your choice of technique would depend on whether or not you were ready to include retention in your practice.

Regulating the breath can also be a powerful tool for managing stress. The body, breath, and mind are the same stuff at different densities or rates of vibration—like ice, water, and steam. The breath is the intermediary level. As such, it is the link between the body and mind. Everything that is happening within, both physically and mentally, is expressed through the flow of the breath. And the reverse is also true: By controlling the breath, we can affect what's happening within.

When faced with stressful situations, we move into a pattern known as chest breathing. Unlike deep diaphragmatic breathing, our breathing tends to become shallow, unsteady, and localized higher in the chest. This pattern is part of the "fight or flight" mechanism. At such times, if we take pause, observe the breath, and then consciously make it slow, steady, and deep as in *dirgha svasam*, we can induce a relaxation response. In a more relaxed state, we will be able to more skillfully deal with the situation at hand.

When stressed, we can also get stuck in that mode of functioning, or side of the brain, that is dominant for us. An experiment was done that demonstrated that when the breath flows through the left nostril, there is an increase in blood flow and electrical activity to the right side of the brain; when it flows through the right nostril, there is a corresponding reaction on the left side of the brain. Given these findings, alternate nostril breathing could potentially be helpful for regaining balance and enabling us to see a fuller range of options in stressful situations.

Intuitively, we know that the breath and mind go together, and employ this principle regularly in daily life. If someone is angry, for example, the breath becomes correspondingly agitated. Our common advice is to tell the person to take a few deep breaths. As the breath becomes slower, deeper, and more regular, the mind, too, calms down.

Because of the correlation between the mind and the breath, regulating the breath figures prominently as preparation for meditation. The best preparation for meditation is *pranayama*: three to five rounds of rapid diaphragmatic breathing, followed by five to ten minutes of alternate nostril breathing. The rapid breathing energizes the system and makes the mind very alert; the alternate breathing then harmonizes and balances the energy. This combination gets the mind into optimal condition to focus well and go deep.

Directing the Breath

Directing the breath is an effective technique for pain management. Simply send the incoming breath to the area of distress and release the pain with the exhalation. Once a young child was nearly hysterical with an intense itching rash. Together, we focused on bringing in cool, soothing air, directing it to all the "itchies," and then sending out the "itchies" with the breath. Within ten minutes, the child was totally calm and went outside to play.

I've had numerous experiences that attest to the benefit of this practice. Years back, I underwent a colonoscopy. I did not wish to have any anesthetic and asked to be positioned so that I could view all the monitors, which displayed heart rate, blood pressure, and oxygen perfusion levels of blood. I asked the doctor what the proper range was for each. Whenever I felt any pain or saw an indicator go out of range, I focused two or three breaths on the problem area, and the situation quickly resolved.

I became so absorbed in this experiment that, at one point, I blurted out, "Far out!" This was followed by the doctor softly intoning, "No, far in." He was so intrigued by my enthusiasm that he offered to extend the tour so that I could see my appendix. As interesting as the experience was, I was eager for it to be over. But not wanting to disappoint him, after a slight hesitation, I was able to agree.

Consider using the breath to cope with any discomfort at your next dentist appointment. Inhale and send the energy of the breath to the painful area. Feel the breath surround, fill, and absorb all the painful sensations. Then, release them with the exhalation. It can work surprisingly well in those trying circumstances.

Whenever you direct your thoughts to an area, you also send the *prana* there. You can use this principle to effect tremendous healing. Sri Gurudev used to say: "All that you need to heal are *prana* and mantra"— divine energy and vibrations.

You can visualize *prana* flowing into the body with the breath. Or, you can visualize *prana* in another form—such as light, sound, fire, or water—and imagine it entering through the top of the head, flowing down the body, going to the area in need, and doing its healing work. For example: you can visualize fire burning up any toxins, or water washing away the impurities. Then, visualize all the problems exiting through the soles of the feet. All forms of touch for health, psychic healing, or distance healing—knowingly or unknowingly—use this principle of mentally directing the *pranic* force.

Observing the Breath

Observing the breath is a wonderful approach for formal meditation and for maintaining peace in daily life. Consider the three levels of our being—body, breath, and mind. The body is mostly the product of the past. The mind fluctuates between the past and future, landing on the present moment intermittently as it whirls about. The breath, however, is always in the now. When we link our attention to the breath, our awareness becomes established in the present moment. We spiral out of control due to memory and anticipation. We can summon an enormous capacity to cope simply by staying in the moment. The mind becomes concentrated and gains power.

There are various ways to meditate on the breath. You can observe the movement of the abdomen, the airflow at the nostrils, the pauses at the bottom of the exhalation and the top of the inhalation, or the corresponding energy movement along the spine. You can listen to the sound of the breath as it flows in and out. Whichever approach you choose, the breath will lead you to a deeper state of awareness and stillness. When the mind becomes very calm, a subtle inner heat is generated. This warmth then awakens the *kundalini*—the storehouse of cosmic *prana* within. Once that is awakened, our consciousness expands; the body, senses, and mind come under our control, culminating in realization of our true nature.

Messages in the Breath

The resounding message of the breath is: connection. The breath is the subtle thread that runs throughout creation. It is our primary connection to life. It connects our inner world with the outer. It is the link between the body and the mind. It is a gateway through which our everyday consciousness can enter higher awareness.

Additionally, the breath can either be voluntary or involuntary. It's as if another message has been encoded in our system, a constant reminder in the flow of the breath, telling us that we have a choice: We can function in an unconscious, involuntary way, or we can exert proper effort and gain control and mastery. In other words, bondage or liberation is in our hands. That is the message that lies hidden in the breath.

Seeing Unity

In bright red letters over the Grand Archway leading to the Light Of Truth Universal Shrine (LOTUS), in Virginia, we boldly proclaim: "Truth is One, Paths are Many." This is a variation of the famous saying from the *Rig Veda*, *"Ekam sat viprah bahudha vadanti,"* which means: "Truth is one; seers express it in many ways." Swami Satchidananda used to say, "Hunger is one, foods are many." Some like spaghetti, others prefer soup, and then there are those who insist upon salad. How silly it would seem if the salad people one day got together and insisted that salad was the only way to satisfy hunger. And what if the spaghetti people challenged them, resulting in a big fight. We would quickly see the foolishness. We know that people have different tastes, temperaments, and capacities. So of course, they would prefer different food.

There is physical hunger, there is also spiritual hunger. When it comes to religion, however, we don't seem to have the same acceptance for people with different inclinations. There is one God who is called by many names such as: Siva, Krishna, Father, Mother, Jesus, Jehovah, Allah, Buddha, or Cosmic Consciousness. Not only do members of different faiths denounce one another, but different groups within the same tradition have problems as well. Shaivites argue with Vaishnavites; Protestants and Catholics come to blows; Sunnis and Shiites vie for power. What to do? What is required is a shift of vision.

Sri Gurudev told a story about a candy shop where he used to go as a young boy. The chocolate was formed into the shapes of various animals. The children would have their favorite animals and be convinced that their candy tasted the best. So, one would think the elephant chocolate was the tastiest, and he would argue with another child who claimed the tiger candy was the most delicious. If they had only understood that it was all the same chocolate made into different shapes, they could have enjoyed the chocolate—the unifying factor— and delighted in the diverse forms without quarreling at all.

The problem is that our ordinary ways of knowing are based not on unity but on discontinuity, both spatial and temporal. This serves as a doorway through which error and illusion can enter. Spatially, there is distance between the observer and the observed, and it is our senses that bridge the gap. Our senses, however, are very limited. We are equipped with only five, and each one can function only within a set range. There is a time lapse, too, as sense data enters through the instrument of perception (such as the eye), and the nerve impulses travel to the brain and are finally understood.

In yogic terms, we say that information is received by the *indriya* (organ of perception), displayed on the *manas* (the recording faculty of the mind) and interpreted by the *buddhi* (the intellect). Then the ego sense, *ahamkara*, "flashes," and somehow we perceive an object in this mix. We are aware of only the end result; we recognize the object. What we perceive are like the dots in a "connect-the-dot" drawing. We see the dots, but the ink that connects them, the underlying process, remains invisible and beyond our grasp.

The master pianist Artur Schnabel once said, "The notes I handle no better than many pianists. But the pauses between the notes—ah, that is where the art resides!" The *Tao Te Ching* states, "We make a vessel from a lump of clay; it is the empty space within the vessel that makes it useful." The beauty, charm, and usefulness depend on what lies beyond ordinary sense perception—that which supports, surrounds, and informs the entire creation. Consider a movie theater. If not for the screen, we wouldn't be able to see the show. But who remembers, who sees, the screen? It is the clear, stable support—the underlying, invisible, unifying factor that makes the show possible. We forget the screen and instead are captivated by the transient images that pass over it. We get caught up in the drama and swept away by the triumphs and tragedies we behold.

Years back, when the first *Star Wars* movie came out, I went to a premiere showing. The theater was packed, the mood electric, and I, a sci-fi aficionado, was primed for the experience. The special effects were amazing, beyond anything ever before seen. The dramatic tension built to a crescendo as the spaceship zoomed into hyperspace for the first time, and I went into hyperspace with them. I leapt onto my seat, threw my arms into the air, and cried out in exultation. In a flash, the entire audience followed suit, all but forgetting that we were just watching a movie, in a theater, in the city of San Francisco. If we could remember the screen, the underlying unity, we would understand the passing images in the proper light. We could fully enjoy the show, without losing our equanimity, balance, and perspective.

Like light shining through cracks, this underlying unity peeks through in the pause between breaths, in the space between thoughts, and in the silence between words. Hindu mythology tells the story of Lord Brahma, the Lord of creation. From his mind were born four sages by name: Sanaka, Sanandana, Sanatana, and Sanatkumara. They wanted to realize the highest truth and sought instruction from God in the form of Dakshinamurti. They humbly prostrated before him, requesting his guidance. He sat there in silence, and in the silence, they had the realization they were seeking. The Hindu scriptures declare: *"OM Mauna vyakhya prakatita parabrahma tattvam"* which means, "The unmanifested supreme principle can only be explained in silence, not by words."

How can we reach that stillness? The paradox is that the path to stillness resides in action. There are three qualities of nature: *sattva,* which represents purity and light; *rajas,* which expresses as passion and action; and *tamas,* which veils the mind in darkness. In order to go from *tamas* to *sattva,* we need to pass through the activity of *rajas.* That is where spiritual practice comes in—all our Hatha Yoga, Raja Yoga, Bhakti Yoga, Karma Yoga, Jnana Yoga, and so on.

Sri Gurudev told the following story. One day, a king decided to visit a temple in his realm. When it came time to distribute the *prasad* (blessed food), he noticed that everyone—the *sadhus,* the devotees, and the servants who worked in the temple—were all given one cake. In the corner, there was a swami just sitting and doing nothing. He didn't even attend the service, but he was also given a cake.

When the king saw that, he demanded, "Who is that fellow? He doesn't seem to be doing anything. Why should he get food? What does he do here?"

The priest gently replied, "Maharaj, he just sits there. We don't know what he is doing. We don't see him doing anything."

So the king went to where the swami was sitting and questioned him, "Are you getting food here daily?"

"Yes, they are giving it to me."

"And what do you do for that?"

"Nothing."

"So you do nothing and you get food?"

"That seems to be what's happening."

"Why should you be given food when you do nothing?"

"Well, Maharaj, it seems to be the most difficult job."

"Ahh, is that so? Well, I can also do nothing."

"Okay, Maharaj, you can try."

So the king sat in front of the swami with his eyes closed for a few minutes, and then announced, "See, I did nothing; it wasn't difficult at all.

"Sir," responded the swami, "please excuse me for saying so, but you were not doing nothing. You were thinking of buying a few more horses for your stables."

Immediately, the king prostrated before the *sadhu*. "Now I understand. Doing nothing doesn't mean simply sitting. The mind also should be totally still, and that is the most difficult thing to achieve." The king turned to the priest and said, "In the future, see that this *sadhu* gets two cakes, not one."

To attain the state of non-doing, we perform a lot of activity in the form of spiritual practice. The *Bhagavad Gita* speaks of finding the action in inaction and the inaction in action. Meditation and Karma Yoga go hand in hand in this process. Through meditation, we discover the action, the inner dynamism, in what might appear to an onlooker as inaction. Through Karma Yoga, we come to understand the inaction, maintaining inner poise, while engaged in outer action. Karma Yoga helps us to step outside our self-created boundaries and embrace others as our very self. Meditation enables us to reduce and ultimately rid ourselves of all the inner noise and clutter. Through both, we are able to eliminate all that limits and partitions our inner space. There's an expansiveness within, and we discover a way to know that transcends the discontinuity inherent in normal sense perception. Our meditation deepens, and we slip into *samadhi*. In that state, there is no longer any separation between subject and object. We experience direct intuitive knowledge.

George Washington Carver, the renowned botanist, explained it this way: "Anything will give up its secrets if you love it enough." In true love, lover and beloved become as one. He would wander the fields in the early morning hours, and the plants would reveal their hidden potential to him. He discovered over three hundred uses for the peanut, and hundreds for the soybean and sweet potato, thereby revolutionizing the field of agriculture.

When we unify the mind by eliminating all its fluctuations, we experience the underlying unity within—the ground of our being, our true Self. When we experience that unity within, we can see it without as well. We see the interconnectedness of all life. With that vision, true humility, compassion, and reverence are born. With that understanding, narrow-mindedness gives way to open-heartedness. Veils of prejudice and intolerance are lifted. We see clearly and become instruments of peace, harmony, and light.

INTEGRATION

Bringing Yoga into Daily Life

Swami Satchidananda used to say, "Yoga is not about learning how to stand on your head; it's about learning how to stand on your feet." He used three words to define Yoga: easeful, peaceful, and useful. If you are easeful in body and peaceful in mind, your life will be useful. By living in that way, you will become fit to realize the higher truth.

Yoga is an attitude, an awareness with which we move through life. Formal practices—*asana, pranayama,* or meditation—are training sessions. We want to bring that same focus, balance, and ease into all that we do. Our entire life then becomes an occasion for spiritual growth and awakening.

We begin by finding a path that resonates with what feels right to us in our hearts. We may be drawn to a particular teacher, a lineage, or a set of wisdom teachings. Then, we follow the practices and techniques that they recommend. At first, our spiritual endeavors may be consigned to specific time slots during the day. At this point, someone might remark, "I did my Yoga today," usually referring to a set of *asanas*, and indicating that the rest of the day was devoted to other activities.

Over time, however, our practice begins to seep into the very fabric of our lives. We start seeing things and responding to situations in new ways. The smallest, most commonplace act becomes an opportunity to practice Yoga; how we perform it is a clear reflection of our level of awareness.

If we really want to make progress, the next step is to consciously cultivate ways to integrate our practice into our lives and to make adjustments, if necessary, so that our lives totally support our practice. When we do this, every moment becomes a meditation; every movement becomes an *asana*. Our spiritual aspirations and our lives become aligned. With proper alignment, we can move efficiently and mindfully toward the goal of Yoga and enjoy health, happiness, and peace in our lives.

Crossing the River of Fire

We're all on the path, right where we are, doing whatever it is that we are doing. The Zen master Dogen observed: "If you cannot find the truth right where you are, where else do you expect to find it?" The path isn't divorced from life; life itself is the path. We are being given the experiences we need to make us fit for the highest realization. Events are perfectly timed and choreographed to enable us to make the next step on our evolutionary journey. That being so, why is it so helpful to deliberately embrace a particular path? Consider "moving sidewalks," those motorized stretches found at airports that facilitate traversing large areas in little time. You can step onto one and just let it carry you to the end. Or, you can walk on it as it moves and feel almost like you are flying. When we consciously apply effort, we accelerate the process. The same is true on the spiritual path.

In the Hindu sacred writings, treading a spiritual path is compared to crossing a bridge made of a single hair suspended over a river of fire. The spiritual path has also been likened to a razor's edge: sharp, straight, and narrow. Similarly, the *Holy Bible* states, "For the gate is small and the way is narrow that leads to life, and there are few who find it." The path is what happens between intention and fulfillment, between aspiration and realization. Success in spiritual life depends on how we handle that gap. It basically comes down to how skillful we are in dealing with five factors: (1) Formal practice; (2) Practice and Daily Life; (3) Obstacles; (4) Commitment; and (5) Support.

Formal Practice

Everywhere in life we see that the higher the goal, the bigger the price. Compare Sunday joggers to Olympic marathon champions. All the joggers need do to prepare is perform a few stretches, select a route, fill their water bottles, and they are set for the afternoon. The Olympians, on the other hand, need to train rigorously many hours a day over many years to get the gold. Self-realization is the highest goal one can attain, so, naturally, it requires the greatest effort.

Effort in spiritual life means discipline. Sometimes, aspirants engage in discipline as if they were complying with rules and restrictions; going to meditation becomes like sitting in detention. If discipline is approached in this way, the mind will undoubtedly resist and eventually rebel. Skillful, successful discipline is not about denial. It's about choosing to embrace practices because your mind is convinced that is the way to true happiness and freedom.

The Sufi mystic, Hafiz, put it this way:

> We should make all spiritual talk
> Simple today:
>
> God is trying to sell you something,
> But you don't want to buy.
>
> That is what your suffering is:
>
> Your fantastic haggling,
> Your manic screaming over the price!

Discipline takes the form of practices to calm and clean the body and mind. Swami Satchidananda states, "Your mind wants to run to its original source of tranquility, but there are impediments on the way that obstruct the flow." The purpose of spiritual practice is to remove these impediments, so we can experience the peace and joy that is our true nature.

To explain this process, Swami Venkatesananda, a brother monk of Sri Gurudev, provides some insightful examples. If you want to see your reflection in a dust-covered mirror, you first need to remove the dust with a cloth. The wiping doesn't create the reflection; the capacity to reflect is in the mirror. But if you don't wipe the mirror, you won't be able to see your face. If you are a gardener and want to grow some plants, you fertilize the soil, sow seeds, and remove any weeds. But you can't make the plant grow; that potential is in the seed. Your job is simply to provide a favorable environment in which the potential of the seed can be manifested.

Wiping the mirror and tending the field correspond to practice. Without them, the mirror's reflective capacity would not be evident, and the plant's potential would not be realized. It may seem like a paradox, but effort is needed in order to realize that which is always present within us as our own true nature. Accordingly, our practices don't bring us enlightenment, but without them, enlightenment won't happen.

For practice to be effective, it needs to be done on a regular, daily basis. Try to have at least two sittings a day for meditation. The best times are before dawn and at dusk. At these junctures between day and night, a peaceful vibration naturally prevails in the atmosphere. If that's not possible, then first thing when you arise in the morning and last thing before you retire.

There are various approaches depending on the taste, temperament, capacity, and beliefs of the aspirant. You can experiment for a while and then choose what appeals to you. Once you've chosen, stick to that and go deep. Otherwise, your very method becomes counter-productive to your goal, which is to make the mind steady and one-pointed. There are many paths to the goal, but if you keep changing, it's tantamount to circling a mountain rather than climbing to the summit.

Practice and Daily Life

Imagine you want to train a puppy, and, given your busy schedule, you decide to devote one hour a day, three days a week to the task. Will that puppy ever get trained? Absolutely not! The same is true with the monkey-mind. You need to be at it constantly. Even if you practice every day for two full hours, but let the mind run amok for the remaining twenty-two, which force will predominate in your life? Clearly, "amok" will be in the lead, eleven to one! The same qualities you would utilize in training a puppy can be applied to your *sadhana* (spiritual practice): patience, perseverance, firmness, loving-kindness, and gentleness. You need to know when to be strict and when to give in; you want to train the mind, not break its spirit.

To have continual practice, you need to find ways to bring the peace, focus and awareness from your formal practice into your daily life. Depending on your chosen method, there are many possibilities to consider. You can silently repeat a mantra as you go about your activities. Or, try to remain as the witness, observing the mind and body as you move through different experiences. If you are devotional, you can cultivate the feeling that God's presence is everywhere, in everyone and everything. You can work on a virtue, like one of the ten ethical precepts, known as *yama-niyama*. You can maintain the spirit of Karma Yoga in all of your actions. Or, just apply throughout the day one of the lessons learned on your Hatha Yoga mat, such as: balance, poise, acceptance, or surrender; knowing when to respect your limits and when to stretch them, when to relax and when to exert.

If you can't keep up this awareness all the time, narrow the field. For example, if you can't feel the divine presence in everyone, pick one person as a start. Try treating the person who pushes all your buttons as a special instrument of the Divine to help you progress on your path. You will likely have a very interesting, if not transformative, experience.

Not only do we need to designate ways to bring practice into our daily activities, but we also need to look at our life and see that it supports our practice. In Raja Yoga, this is described as practice and non-attachment; both are needed for the mind to retain its peace. Through practice, we strengthen the body and mind, and eliminate any toxins and tensions in the system. In the name of non-attachment, we avoid those activities that cause the problems in the first place. If our lifestyle doesn't reflect our beliefs, our everyday endeavors and our spiritual practice will pull us in opposite directions. Confusion and conflict—both within and without—may ensue.

See that everything you allow in through the gateways of the senses is conducive to the health of the body and a pure, balanced state of mind. You are what you eat, and you eat through all the senses. Look at your food, music, movies, books, possessions, associations, etc. Look, also, at the types of thoughts you regularly entertain. If you get into negative patterns, make an effort to turn them around. You can't expect to experience the light if you cling to the darkness in the form of anger, jealousy, or resentment. Every little thought is a seed that has the capacity to grow into a great tree and bear fruit if we water it by repetition.

Even athletes training for the Olympics need to watch their diet, make lifestyle adjustments and schedule all their other activities to support this primary goal. Imagine if you want to fill a jar with large rocks, small rocks, sand, and water. You would need to put the big items in first. Otherwise, there won't be room for them after the other items are put in place. Similarly, if you are dedicated to your spiritual path, your practice needs to be a "big rock" that you prioritize in your life. Otherwise, the seeming urgency and preponderance of other concerns could easily preempt your time.

Obstacles

Life is a grand obstacle race in which we continually face challenges in pursuit of our goals. From the very beginning, conception itself, this point is made very clear. Millions of sperm rush toward one goal: fertilizing the egg. Some get bottlenecked, exhausted, confused, turned around, or are just too weak to make the journey. But the good news is that one champion who succeeds, that hero, is you. You're one in a million. From the outset, you've proven that you have what it takes to overcome tremendous obstacles and attain your goal.

Obstacles aren't bad. They goad us to take action. They impel us to tap new resources—both inner and outer—that otherwise we may never have known we had. They can set us on a new trajectory of growth and development, and enable us to manifest our potential in fuller and more fulfilling ways. They can lead us to deeper levels of faith, acceptance and surrender. Obstacles represent our growing edge, where our character may need to be strengthened, our intellect sharpened, our talents honed or our heart softened. Seen in this light, obstacles are not "in the way;" they "are the way." They help to mold and refine us, preparing us for the highest realization.

I once spoke with Swami Satchidananda about making progress on the spiritual path. He said if you were to chart someone's path, it would never look like a line going straight upward, because no one ever goes right to the goal. There are always challenges and lessons to learn. Instead, the graph would more closely resemble a line gently sloping upward, with intervals of spiraling up and down along the way.

To stay the course on such a journey requires a balance between exertion and surrender, knowing when to actively confront an impediment and when to just let it be. Sri Gurudev used to say: "We need to take it easy, but not lazy. We need to do our best and then leave the rest." The "Serenity Prayer" of Reinhold Niebuhr provides this wise counsel: "God grant me the serenity to accept the things I cannot change, the courage to change the things I can, and the wisdom to know the difference."

There is also a difference between affirming and demanding. Affirming opens and attunes us to receive the energy and support we need to face any challenge. It aligns us with the subtle principle: As you think, so you become. It paves the way for a solution to unfold. Demanding, on the other hand, entails an unspoken ultimatum that our way is the only acceptable solution. There is an undercurrent of impatience, if not antagonism, toward the problem we are facing. Demanding is constricting; it obstructs us from seeing other options or recognizing the gifts that the obstacle may be bestowing in the form of lessons learned, karma purged, and new connections made.

In dealing with an obstacle, the following method can be effective. First, explore if there are any outer adjustments you can make to help rectify the situation. Next, consider if there are any inner adjustments, like a shift in attitude that could prove useful. Then, formulate an implementation plan. This can include designating progressive steps, setting a timeline, or enlisting the aid of others. Finally, establish a clear way to monitor your progress. Personal accountability in the form of a spiritual diary is a powerful tool to help stay on track. Daily review and recording of what is transpiring can provide insight as to the inner workings of your process and can shed light on what remains to be done. It can also be a source of inspiration and motivation when you see charted before you all the progress that has been made.

If you keep on practicing, obstacles will yield to your persistence like water wearing down a mountain of granite. You will have greater clarity to find good solutions. And as you become stronger, what may have seemed like an impediment before will no longer trouble you at all.

Commitment

Commitment is crucial, not only to the goal, but to the journey. The author Ursula Le Guin once said, "It is good to have an end to journey toward, but it is the journey that matters in the end." Many seekers affirm commitment to the goal, but they give up because they don't want to deal with the process. We are like gold being purified. Lots of crude ore has to be removed to uncover a single nugget of precious gold. Then, to refine the gold further, it has to be heated and cooled numerous times. Just think of what a simple piece of soiled linen has to undergo to become clean and useful again. It has to be washed well with detergent, placed in a hot dryer, and then all the wrinkles have to be ironed out. It's a painful process no doubt, but necessary to recover the initial beauty of the cloth. Likewise, as Sri Gurudev often explained, we were fine originally, and now we have to "re-fine" ourselves.

Without commitment, it's hard to stay on track. We might think that something we're doing is only a little bit off course, a small detour, but even a small angle of difference will result in us winding up far from our destination. People more often lose their way through little things that take them bit by bit off course, than by some major flaw which is obvious for all to see, and they're on guard against. It's the little things that make or break our spiritual edifice. Franz Kafka once noted, "The true way goes over a rope which is not stretched at any great height, but just above the ground. It seems more designed to make people stumble than to be walked upon."

Commitment is like a walking stick that helps steady us through all the twists and turns on the path. It serves as a shield against wily assailants, like boredom, restlessness, distractions, excuses, and inner resistance. It changes your relationship to your practice. Consider what happens when you make a commitment in a personal relationship. The relationship becomes a priority in your life, and you invest even more time and energy into making it work. This type of dedication is essential on the spiritual path. We need to walk purposefully, effectively, and efficiently. This is possible only if our efforts are backed by unwavering commitment, and as Sri Gurudev would urge, we stop not till the goal is reached.

Support

Positive change is difficult; so many forces pull us in other directions. Just like a tender plant needs a protective fence till it grows strong, new aspirants need support to help them get established in a steady practice. Longtime seekers, too, need support, because for them, the tests get harder. Sri Gurudev used to say, "Trust and test go together. The more you trust God, the more you are tested." Even Mother Teresa remarked, "I know God won't give me anything I can't handle. I just wish he didn't trust me so much."

We can access guidance and support through prayer, study, and connecting with one another. The *Holy Bible* clearly states: "Ask and it shall be given you; seek and ye shall find; knock and it shall be opened unto you." The entire universe is there to support us on our spiritual quest. A scripture or sacred text that is read regularly becomes like a trusted friend and guide. When you turn to it with a prayerful heart, it has a way of providing exactly what you need to hear at that moment. We can find helpful guidance in books, CDs, DVDs, and on the Internet. By playing mantras, we can imbue our environment with spiritual vibrations. Paramahansa Yogananda used to say, "Environment is stronger than willpower." A spiritually charged environment is a tremendous aid toward maintaining our clarity of intention and regularity in practice.

Spiritual centers where seekers practice together provide a wonderful support system for spiritual growth. By visiting such centers, taking retreats and programs, our spiritual batteries get recharged. It's also very helpful to have someone with whom you check in regularly: a teacher, mentor, spiritual buddy, or a group. That way, you can receive individualized feedback and encouragement as your journey unfolds.

Sri Gurudev was fond of quoting a verse from Adi Shankaracharya as to the value of support: *"Satsangatve nissangatvam. Nissangatve nirmohatvam. Nirmohatve nishchalatattvam. Nishchalatattve jivanmuktih."* This translates as: "If you are in good company, you are not in bad company. If you are not in bad company, your mind will not be deluded. If your mind is not deluded, it will be steady. If your mind is steady, you will attain liberation." Just keeping good company initiates a chain reaction that culminates in liberation. That is the beauty and gift of *sangha,* and the purpose of spiritual centers.

We are trying to cross a turbulent river. Alone, we may falter. But together, each of us doing our part and supporting one another along the way, we can cross the river of fire and abide in true peace and joy.

Why Am I Here?

"Why am I here?" Probably most of us at some point along the way have stopped and pondered some version of this question. What is my purpose in life? Why do I find myself in these particular circumstances? Is there a deeper meaning behind my existence? Is there a reason the world is the way it is, and do I have a role in some overall plan?

These are points for profound reflection and can be addressed on many levels. Let's begin with the events that precede a given birth. At the time of death, the soul is churned to its depths. Of all the desires still awaiting fulfillment, the strongest comes to the top and sets the course for the next birth. So, the first answer to our question is: We are here because we still have desires to be satisfied. Desire is what propels us onward from birth to birth.

According to the yogic teachings, the soul then looks for a favorable environment, one that will provide the experiences it needs to continue on its evolutionary journey. In this way, the soul selects the family into which it will be born. We have no one to blame for our family situation, because on a subtle level, we ourselves chose it. Years ago, I was speaking with a child at Satchidananda Ashram in Virginia whose parents were going through a divorce. Even at her tender age, she recognized that her parents weren't right for one another, and at the same time, she was certain they were both perfect for her.

Such insight is the sign of an evolved soul. Swami Satchidananda told us that the children who lived at the *ashram* were *yogabrashtas*, souls who had practiced Yoga in their previous birth, but had not attained the final goal. The *Bhagavad Gita* states that such individuals will take their next birth either in a pure and prosperous home or one of wise yogis. In such settings, they will have the facilities and support to continue on the yogic path with little delay.

The particular circumstances that we find ourselves in are further determined by our karma, our thoughts and actions from the past that are bearing fruit now, as well as the new thoughts and actions that we are performing. Invisible threads of karma draw to us people, positions, possessions, and all sorts of situations as we move through life. The *Tirukkural* states that, "What is not destined to be yours will not stay even if you guard it; what is destined to be yours will not leave even if you cast it aside."

Our search for a building to house the New York Integral Yoga Institute is an excellent example of the workings of destiny. We finally found the ideal location, but we did not have the funds for a down payment. As the final days were approaching for signing the contract, the person who was overseeing the purchase came to Sri Gurudev a bit distraught, not knowing what to do. Gurudev calmly replied, "If it's meant to be ours, the money will come."

On the very last day, Gurudev was visited by Alice Coltrane, a student and close friend. (She later took monastic vows and was known as Swamini Turiyasangitananda.) They met for a while, and then she left. When she reached the taxi, she realized she had left her checkbook behind. She went back to the Institute to retrieve it. She told Gurudev that she was going to send a donation, but probably this was a sign that she should give him the check now. Gurudev graciously received it and then happily told the fellow, "Sign the contract; we have the money." Over the years, thousands upon thousands of seekers have learned about Yoga there. It has been a beacon of hope, a sanctuary, a residence, a place to serve for many, many people whose lives have been forever transformed thanks to the destiny that secured that building for the IYI.

Our thoughts and actions not only attract our outer environment, they also determine our inner nature and abilities. Swami Sivananda, in speaking about karma, says that if we performed virtuous deeds in our past life, we will find ourselves in a good environment in the current one. If we were charitable in the past, we will be wealthy now. Strong thoughts in our past birth manifest as our character in the current one; our tendencies become capacities. Selfless activities bear the fruit of discrimination, dispassion, and spiritual aspiration.

In this way, each one of us comes equipped with unique talents and experiences that make us ideally suited for certain roles in life. We have our *svadharma*, our own duty to fulfill. Sometimes people wonder what they are supposed to be doing—what their purpose is. Just look at your capabilities and the sorts of activities and opportunities that come naturally to you, and let your work be an expression of that. If it is righteous, if it brings benefit to someone and harm to no one, then that is your *svadharma*.

We needn't compare ourselves with others. We are all here for a purpose and have an essential contribution to make. The *Bhagavad Gita* declares that, "It is better to do your own *dharma* even imperfectly than someone else's perfectly." We have been prepared for that and, if it is going to change, that will happen naturally. Sometimes, boredom, envy, or pride may prompt us to look for something else before we are ready for a new undertaking. All the roles are necessary on the world stage. The measure of our success depends on how well we play our part, and not on the part itself. When the Academy Award is given for the best actor of the year, the Oscar may go to the man who played a butler, rather than to the one who played a king.

This brings us to the ultimate level of inquiry: Who is directing the show and why was this particular screenplay selected? In other words, how was the universe created and why does it exist in its present form? Where did we all come from; why are we here? This has been the query of philosophers, scientists, artists, and theologians throughout the ages. Gaughin's famous triptych is a striking example, the themes being: Where Do We Come From? What Are We? Where Are We Going? This path of inquiry always brings us to the gate of mystery. Great thinkers and mystics have presented different stories in their attempts to convey their insights and revelations.

One explanation, from a devotional perspective, is that we are here because God got bored. Everywhere God looked, all God saw was God. There was no one else to play with. So the One multiplied itself and became many, and the games began. If you have a sheet of plain cardboard, you can't play. But if you cut it up and draw different pictures on the pieces, you have a deck of cards, and there are innumerable games to play. The purpose behind the game of life is for the many to rediscover the One. After experiencing the pangs of separation, the individual soul experiences the bliss of union with God. In other words, God creates the illusion of duality in order to experience the joy of love.

Sri Gurudev used to say, "A lifetime is like a flash in the pan. Don't waste this one in trivial pursuits. Do everything you can to realize God. You don't know when you will get this opportunity again." Adi Shankaracharya, one of India's greatest philosophers, said there are three great blessings one can have: The first is a human birth, because it is only in a human birth that one can realize the truth. The second is the thirst for the truth, and the third is association with great souls, so you will receive the proper guidance to attain it. Sri Gurudev said if you have all three, "Make hay while the sun shines." We don't know when all three will converge on our path again.

Such opportunities come as the result of prayer, penance, and good deeds done in the past. We don't know how long we will have the health, strength, clarity, and opportunity to pursue the highest goal. The *Tirukkural* compares a life to a tree. A day is like an axe cutting a nick in the tree. We never know when the last critical cut will be made, and the tree of our life will come tumbling down.

Several months before his *Mahasamadhi,* his passage from this earthly plane, Sri Gurudev was talking to a few senior members. He was recalling his early days with the American devotees, how inspired he was by the intensity of our longing for the highest realization. We were on fire for God, and there was no sacrifice too great, no task too challenging, that we wouldn't embrace it in a heartbeat.

At the San Francisco Integral Yoga Institute, our members served seven days a week. There were no answering machines, and I can remember the concerned discussions that took place when we first considered using them, lest they compromise the quality of our service. Wakeup was at 4 a.m., and the day ended with evening meditation at 9 p.m. That was the type of energy and dedication that laid the foundation and built the IYI into one of the most respected Yoga organizations in the world.

How many of us can honestly say that we approach our spiritual life now with the same fervor as when we first embarked on our spiritual path? The *Yoga Sutras* lists "slipping from ground gained" as a major obstacle on the spiritual path. We slip in little ways. We get a little lazy in our practices. Maybe substances or activities we once abandoned slowly creep back into our life. We begin to forget in little ways, and this forgetfulness is *maya's* trap. Each time we make a choice contrary to our higher good, she clutches us more firmly in her grasp.

So, how can we keep the flame of aspiration burning bright? We can inspire one another by our commitment to the teachings, our personal practice, and our example. We can support one another through the joys and sorrows that every path encompasses. That is what *sangha* is all about. *Sangha* is not limited to a physical location. The *Tirukkural* notes that, "Frequent meetings and constant association are not necessary; it is mutual feeling only which gives the privilege of friendship." We can link up through prayer and practice, through remembrance and intention.

We are here. Desire, karma, *dharma*, and ultimately, a Higher Power, have all come together to fashion the special gift that is our life. So, let's make the most of this precious opportunity. Let each revolution around the sun be a celebration of greater love, light, peace, and joy in our hearts and in our lives.

Laying a Strong Foundation

It was September 1970 when I first met Swami Satchidananda. The place was Camp Kennolyn, a rustic site in the Santa Cruz Mountains. Several hundred of us had gathered there for our first spiritual retreat. We were eager, searching, and receptive. In the cool mountain air, we sat rapt in an atmosphere electric with wisdom and power and permeated with profound peace and love. On those five precious days, Sri Gurudev presented the teachings of Raja Yoga and changed my life forever. As he spoke, tears began to flow. I had spent my college years seeking answers through science and philosophy and had graduated with even more questions. Finally, I was hearing answers to all my questions, and in a way that resonated with my own inner knowing. For the first time that I could recall, my mind became quiet and knew peace.

The retreat became an annual event and, the following year, Sri Gurudev spoke at length on *yama* and *niyama*, the first two limbs of Sri Patanjali's eight-limbed system of Raja Yoga. *Yama* refers to the Great Vows, certain abstinences that all are enjoined to follow. It includes: *ahimsa* (non-violence), *satya* (truthfulness), *asteya* (non-stealing), *brahmacharya* (continence), and *aparigraha* (non-greed). Patanjali says these vows are universal—for all people, in all cultures, at all times. They are reflected in five of the Ten Commandments: Thou shalt not kill, bear false witness, steal, commit adultery, or covet thy neighbor's wife or possessions. They are moral precepts that prohibit certain behaviors. *Niyama* refers to certain observances, standards for spiritual life: *saucha* (purity), *santosha* (contentment), *tapas* (accepting pain as help for purification), *svadhyaya* (spiritual study), and *Ishvara pranidhana* (surrender to God). Together, they comprise the ethical foundation of Yoga.

Their paramount importance soon became clear. Our goal is to make the mind calm and clean. Such a mind is like a crystal clear lake; we can see to its depths and experience our true divine nature. If we disregarded *yama* and *niyama*, it would be impossible to keep the mind serene. Violence, lying, greed, and the rest would darken and agitate the mental landscape. If we ignored *yama* and *niyama* and rushed to pursue higher states of consciousness, not only would our efforts be futile, but harm could ensue.

We might succeed in focusing the mind for a while by dint of concentrated effort, but without ethical purity, we would not be able to sustain that state. More importantly, we could prematurely awaken the *kundalini shakti*, the subtle energy within. Once that energy is released, whatever is in the mind gains tremendous power. All the tendencies are magnified. A small weakness now could become an all-consuming addiction. Any negative traits would be even more troublesome for others—and for us as well—as we faced the karmic consequences of our actions. The safer path is to let the energy awaken naturally as a result of a life of purity. This comes through the observance of *yama* and *niyama* and by being regular in our spiritual practice.

Realizing all this, I left the retreat with a resolve to spend the next year working on *yama* and *niyama*, focusing on one a month. I was a typical beginner: zealous, but clueless as to my capacity. The first one was *ahimsa*, so I decided to be non-violent in thought, word, and deed. Sri Gurudev had spoken about setting a consequence if you slip as a very effective method when trying to accomplish spiritual goals. The consequence could be any beneficial practice—like another set of *asanas*, spiritual study, or more meditation. But being a beginner, I chose what seemed to be most challenging: If I failed in my resolve, I would fast for the entire day.

Needless to say, my lower mind was equal to the challenge. Normally, I would only have what could be considered a violent thought on very rare occasions—if I were frustrated or angry over a situation. But now, on many a day, my mind would manufacture such a thought shortly after arising, and I would have to fast for the rest of the day. This became somewhat unnerving, but since I had sent Sri Gurudev a note telling him of my resolve, I persevered.

A year passed, much was learned, and I decided to have a second go-around with all the precepts. There was my old friend, *ahimsa*.

But by now, I was a more seasoned aspirant. Whereas before, my goal was to be non-violent in thought, word, and deed, now it was simply to set a goal such that I would be able to eat every day. So, I eliminated trying to control my thoughts; that would be too hard. Then I eliminated trying to control speech. Even being vigilant with respect to all actions seemed too taxing. So, I kept narrowing the field till, at last, I came to: doors. In the name of *ahimsa*, I wouldn't slam doors.

This was a moment of stark personal reckoning. I thought I could be totally established in non-violence, only to discover that there was no guarantee that I would even close a door gently. But that month spent trying not to slam doors turned out to be one of the most important spiritual exercises of my life. It laid the foundation for all the inner work I've done ever since.

It was meaningful on two counts. First, it addressed the level I was at. Previously, I had been trying to fly, when I was just learning to crawl. No real growth can happen under such circumstances. And second, spiritual practice became integrated into my daily life, no longer confined to a couple of hours at the beginning and end of the day. We walk through doors continually throughout the day, and each time I did, it was a reminder to become totally present. And not only that, my vision expanded: I began to see doors everywhere. A sliding window was a door, a lid for a box became a door, even a zipper was a door of sorts. This greater insight then went on to inform my practice of the other virtues as well.

I would begin each month by reading about the precept in various scriptures, like the *Yoga Sutras*, *Tirukkural*, *Bhagavad Gita*, and *Bible*, so I could understand it better. Then, I would study the lives of people who embodied it. For *ahimsa*, there was St. Francis, the Buddha, and Mahatma Gandhi. Gandhi's *satyagraha* movement that secured the independence of India was predicated on the first two precepts: *ahimsa* and *satya*. For *satya*, I based my practice on a *sloka* from the *Bhagavad Gita* that describes discipline of speech as: non-agitating, truthful, pleasant, and beneficial. If what I was going to say didn't meet all four criteria, I tried to rephrase it or just remained silent. I spent one week on each quality and then a fifth week practicing all of them together. Needless to say, the fifth week I was very quiet. Since speech is a major way we relate to one another, I learned a lot about communication, social interaction, and by speaking less and listening more, what the real message behind the words often was. And so my practice of these precepts continued. Through personal experience, I learned much more than any books or lectures could convey.

One thing I learned was that I could fashion my spiritual practice so that the progress I was making became visible. Have you ever felt that even though you practice every day, you don't see much progress on your path? Here's a way to turn that around. You can create exercises for yourself that take you step by step toward fulfilling your goals. That way, the mind gains confidence, sees the progress, and builds on success. I call it "designer spirituality," rather than a "one size fits all" approach. The hints given below provide a guide for designing spiritual exercises.

Helpful Hints for Practicing *Yama* and *Niyama*

1. *Goal Setting:* Honestly evaluate your capacity. Then, be specific and practical in setting a goal. Make your goal challenging, but attainable; if you apply proper effort, you will succeed. If you make it too hard, you will only set yourself up for frustration and failure, and give your mind an excuse to give up. Beware of this trick of the mind that can sabotage your progress. Don't let the subtle machinations of pride entice you to reach too far, too fast. Slow and steady wins the race. Even if you are focusing on what may seem like a small, mundane thing, what you're really doing is cultivating greater awareness that can then express in other areas of your life.

   Designate a consequence in case you slip. Let it be another beneficial practice: like more *pranayama*, meditation, service, study, or a dietary observance. That way, you will be continually asserting your mastery over the mind. Be creative; make it fun. Lovingly, patiently, skillfully win over any inner resistance, so that your mind becomes your ally, rather than an adversary in this process.

2. *Positive Affirmations*: State what you wish to develop clearly and succinctly. If you practice mantra *japa*, repeat your affirmation several times before the silent repetition of your mantra. When you do that, the power of the mantra goes to fulfill the intention behind your affirmation. It's also very helpful to repeat the affirmation several times upon arising and before retiring at night. The first thing you do in the morning makes a deep impression in the mind that will influence the rest of the day. By repeating it again before sleep, it slips into the subconscious mind. That way, you will be continually integrating the virtue you are developing into your character and expressing it more and more in your life.

3. *Pratipaksha Bhavana:* This yogic technique helps to overcome negative patterns by consciously cultivating the opposite positive ones. It can be combined with alternate nostril breathing. As you inhale, visualize that along with the breath, you are drawing into yourself the positive quality you wish to develop. Feel like it is filling you completely. When you exhale, visualize that the negative pattern is leaving with the breath. While it's difficult to change personality habits directly, this single technique can help a lot in this regard. Because it is so simple and mechanical, it bypasses the mind's resistance and defenses. Analogously, in the original *Star Wars* movie, the Death Star was fortified to withstand a major attack, but totally vulnerable to a single fighter plane, because they didn't expect a small thing to be so powerful. According to Swami Sivananda, it takes twenty-one days to build a new habit. Try practicing this technique twice a day for ten minutes, for a month, and see the benefits.

4. *Inspiration:* Find out more about others who embody the virtue you're developing. You can draw examples from the saints and sages of the various faith traditions or from leaders in different fields, such as: government, public service, science, technology, business, sports, or the arts. If you look around you, you will also be able to draw inspiration from family members, colleagues, community members, teachers, students, and friends. Seeing the virtue active in others can help make your goal seem more accessible; seeing all the benefits that come when it is expressed

in their lives can serve as a powerful motivator to strive more ardently yourself.

5. *Personal Accountability:* Every day, pause, reflect, and record your progress in a spiritual journal. A few moments a day in this way will help to keep you on track and deepen your spiritual discernment. A greater understanding of the meaning, benefits, and power of the virtue you are developing will be revealed to you.

6. *Support:* This is very important when you set out to achieve higher goals. You can draw support from the Higher Power through prayer and sincere, heartfelt efforts. You can also draw support from fellow aspirants. This can be a source of valuable feedback as your practice deepens.

May you practice well, enjoy the benefits, and then share them with one and all.

All About Action

Did you ever try to do nothing? I have, and it's harder than you might think. Just try this experiment. Say to yourself, "I am not going to do anything," and see how long that lasts. Within seconds, you will probably find yourself pursuing a line of thought or moving about. Within minutes, you may have forgotten the exercise altogether, as bodily needs or life's obligations hijacked your attention.

We are made to act. The forces of nature—*sattva, rajas,* and *tamas*—are always in flux. Our bodies and minds, as part of nature, are subject to these changes. We are continually interacting with our environment—breathing, eating, speaking, moving, working, playing—engaging in the myriad activities of life. The *Bhagavad Gita* declares, "Perfection in action is Yoga." Skillful action can pave the way for both worldly success and spiritual attainment. Great thinkers and spiritual luminaries throughout the ages have provided insightful keys toward this end.

Albert Einstein was guided by "Three Rules of Work": (1) Out of clutter, find simplicity. (2) From discord, find harmony. (3) In the middle of difficulty lies opportunity. Rule #1 would be no less helpful to someone organizing a desk or prioritizing a schedule than it would be to the brilliant scientist who intuited the grand laws at the foundation of the universe. Rule #2 could be well applied in our homes, at work, among followers of different faiths, and between nations. Rule #3 would be good advice for anyone facing a challenge. We can see this principle exemplified by another great thinker when faced with a crisis in his life.

In 1914, when Thomas Edison was sixty-seven years old, his laboratory was practically destroyed by fire. The buildings were insured for only a fraction of the cost of the damage. The next day, gazing at the ruins, Edison calmly stated, "There is a great value in disaster. All our mistakes are burned up. Thank God we can start anew." Edison listed three great essentials for achieving anything worthwhile: (1) Hard work, (2) Stick-to-itiveness, and (3) Common sense. He is credited with stating, "Genius is one percent inspiration and ninety-nine percent perspiration."

The importance and power of skillful action is explored in the *Tirukkural*, the preeminent scripture of South India. One verse poses the question, "Are there any impossible deeds, if one does them by suitable means after finding out the suitable time to do them?" And the next one asserts, "Even if a person were to think of ruling the whole world, he will succeed if he ascertains the proper time and acts at the strategic place." Keys to skillful action and the importance of timing are also echoed in the ancient Taoist scripture, the *Tao Te Ching:*

In cultivating your mind, know how to dive in the hidden deeps.
In dealing with others, know how to be gentle and kind.
In speaking, know how to keep your words.
In governing, know how to maintain order.
In transacting business, know how to be efficient.
In making a move, know how to choose the right moment.

Both scriptures give similar advice on how to deal with failure. The *Tirukkural* cautions: "Most people give up on the verge of success." The *Tao Te Ching* goes further and states: "In handling affairs, people often spoil them just at the point of success. With heedfulness in the beginning and patience at the end, nothing will be spoiled."

The value of this advice is beautifully exemplified in the life of Robert Bruce, a heroic king of Scotland. According to legend, he was defeated in battle six times. Having lost everything, he fled and hid in a cave. He had abandoned all hope when he noticed a spider trying to spin a web. The first step was to affix a central thread from the ground to the roof. The spider jumped, but missed the roof and fell down. Six times it tried and failed, just like him. Then, with one mighty leap, it accomplished its goal.

Watching the efforts of the spider, the king reflected, "If a little spider can have that kind of perseverance and ultimately succeed, why can't I do the same?" He put aside his despair, re-gathered his troops, and was victorious. Thus, Scotland won its independence from England, and Robert Bruce was recognized as its king.

Swami Satchidananda enjoined us to have that type of resilient determination in life. He boldly said: "Never, never, never give up. Don't have the word 'impossible' in your dictionary. Everything is possible. That should be our attitude in spiritual practice." The *Yoga Sutras of Patanjali* includes failure to reach firm ground and slipping from the ground gained as typical obstacles on the spiritual path and adds that they may be accompanied by distress and despair. Knowing that this is common on the path and that many others have experienced similar challenges should help fortify us if ever we face a slippery slope ourselves.

Life sometimes can feel like an obstacle course where we're negotiating hurdles, racing others to attain some coveted end: it could be a position, a promotion, placement at a chosen school, or the affection of a potential partner or spouse. Very often this spirit of competition is fraught with frustration, anxiety, and disappointment. Competition is the first level of action. From there, we evolve to cooperation—the mutual sharing and exchange of our gifts and goods with others. We work together for a common purpose. A higher level still is dedication—giving all that we have without thought of receiving anything in return. This is when action becomes truly skillful. It is here that we touch the Divine.

Years ago, at a Special Olympics in Seattle, nine children participated in the 100-yard dash. They were all physically or mentally challenged, but they had trained for the event, and each one was eager to win. Shortly after the race began, one of the children fell and started to cry. The other children stopped in their tracks, turned around, and went back to comfort their "opponent." They gently helped him to his feet and then, with one mind (or rather, one heart), they linked arms and walked the track together. As they crossed the finish line, the crowd jumped to their feet for a standing ovation. Competition had yielded to dedication, to loving and giving above all else, and everyone present recognized that they were witnessing something extraordinary.

Mother Teresa said, "Small things with great love: It is not how much we do, but how much love we put into doing it; and it is not how much we give, but how much love we put in the giving. To God, there is nothing small. The moment we have given it to God, it becomes infinite." Thomas Jefferson would most certainly concur: "He does most in God's great world who does his best in his own little world."

Brother Lawrence, well known for his teaching on practicing the presence of God, echoes this same wisdom:

"And it is not necessary to have great things to do.... I turn over my little omelet in the frying pan for the love of God. When it is finished, if I have nothing to do, I prostrate myself on the ground and adore my God from whom the grace came to make it. After that, I get back up, more content than a king. When I cannot do anything else, it is enough for me to have picked up a straw from the ground for the love of God.

"People search for methods...to learn to love God. They wish to arrive at it by I do not know how many practices. They make painful attempts to remain in the presence of God by a multitude of methods. Is it not much shorter and more direct to do everything for the love of God, to use every one of our duties to show that love to Him, and to maintain His presence in us by the communion of our hearts with Him?"

"The time of business," he used to say, "is no different from the time of prayer. I possess God as tranquilly in the noise and clatter of my kitchen, where sometimes several people ask me different things at the same time, as if I were on my knees before the Blessed Sacrament." Sri Gurudev spoke of the same experience when he said, "Work is worship."

Ultimately, it's all about action. From the moment of conception till our final expiration, life's momentum propels us onward. Action performed skillfully, lovingly, mindfully ensures success in our everyday endeavors and paves the way for the highest spiritual attainment as well.

Enlightened Eating

The ancient yogis noted that the universe goes through cycles of potentiality and manifestation, similar to the speculations of modern-day physicists about an oscillating universe. During the process of creation, out of primordial matter known as undifferentiated *Prakriti*, everything evolves—from the mind itself, to the subtle and gross elements, to the world, as we know it.

Swami Vivekananda observed that, "In this universe, there is one continuous substance on every plane of existence. Physically, this universe is one." Swami Satchidananda used to say, "We are interdependent, cells of one universal body." The 17th century English poet, John Donne, expressed the same truth: "No man is an island, entire of itself; every man is a piece of the continent, a part of the main. If a clod be washed away by the sea, Europe is the less, as well as if a promontory were, as well as if a manor of thy friend's or of thine own were. Any man's death diminishes me, because I am involved in mankind; and therefore never send to know for whom the bell tolls; it tolls for thee."

All life is interconnected, and from there arises the beauty, elegance, and mystery in the divine plan of creation. Survival depends on mutual support, enlightened stewardship, and sacrifice. Sri Gurudev often noted that sacrifice is the law of life. The candle sacrifices to give us light; the incense stick to provide fragrance; the apple tree offers its fruits for all to enjoy. The *Bhagavad Gita* explains, "After creating humanity together with *yajna* (sacrifice), the Creator said, 'Through sacrifice you will increase yourself and get everything that you want.'" Even rain, it declares, is the result of sacrifice, and from rain comes food and all beings. When there is sacrifice, the elements become favorable toward us and bless the earth with abundance.

The need to eat is at the basis of survival and is fundamental to the design and functioning of every society. It is a determining factor in our economic systems. It defines many of our cultural norms for social interaction. The choices we make as to how, when, where, and what we eat have great impact on our personal spiritual growth, as well as on the delicate balance of life on our planet.

There is a story in the *Mahabharata*, the great religious epic from India, which Sri Gurudev used to tell that illustrates some of these points. It describes an episode in the life of the noble Pandava family. Once Yudhisthira, the eldest brother, decided to conduct a great *yajna* (ritual sacrifice). In the midst of the ceremonies, a strange-looking mongoose suddenly appeared and began rolling in the remnants of the food that had been offered. Then it stood up, examined its body, and looked quite disappointed.

Clearly, this was not an ordinary mongoose. Aside from its peculiar behavior, one half of its body was a beautiful golden color. So Yudhisthira asked the mongoose for an explanation.

"I used to be an ordinary mongoose, without this golden color," the mongoose recounted. "One day, during a time of great famine, I was very hungry. I came upon a small hut, where a poor teacher, his wife, their son, and daughter-in-law lived. Fortunately, one of the teacher's students had brought them a little flour for bread. The wife prepared four *rotis* (wholemeal Indian bread), one for each of them. When everything was ready, the teacher came out of the house and looked around to see if anybody was coming.

"The scriptures say: *'Atithi devo bhavah,'* which means 'treat the guest as God.' It is the custom of pious people at mealtime to go outside the house and see if there is anyone passing by who is hungry. They would be fed first, and if there were anything left over, then the family would eat. The teacher saw somebody approaching, so he invited him to dine.

"The teacher, his wife, the son, and daughter-in-law all came forward in turn and offered their portions to the guest, who graciously accepted the bread. After eating everything, the guest blessed the family and left. The poor family collapsed and died of hunger, but their faces were radiant with joy.

"Because I was so hungry, I checked to see if there were any crumbs left. There were a few on the floor, not really fit for eating, so I just rolled in them. When I got up, I saw that half of my body had become golden, so I thought something extraordinary must have happened here. Then I realized these people had performed a holy *yajna;* they had sacrificed themselves for the sake of another.

"Since then, I've been traveling all over trying to make the other half of my body golden. When I heard that the Pandavas were performing a grand royal *yajna,* I came running. I rolled in the remnants, but nothing has changed. It seems the humble gift of bread by that family, at the cost of their own lives, was a greater offering."

The *Tirukkural,* a great scripture from South India, proclaims: "Is it even necessary to sow in the field of one who eats the food left over after feeding guests?" In life, we are meant to love and give, care and share. If we live this way, in accordance with nature's law, there is food enough for everyone. Just like milk is produced in the breast of the mother when a baby is developing in her womb, so, too, nature will provide enough food for everyone. Again, the *Tirukkural* states: "Seasonal rains, together with unlimited produce, are found in the realm of the ruler who wields his scepter justly." The elements, themselves, respond to our thoughts, words, and deeds. Consciousness is everywhere, and all life is interconnected.

Even in the face of survival, we are called to rise above selfishness, to share, to sacrifice, and to cause as little pain as possible. No matter what we eat, something offers itself to become a part of and nourish us. Life requires the sacrifice of life in order to continue. Even plucking a carrot from the earth no doubt causes pain to the plant. But as spiritual seekers, we can choose to cause as little pain as possible by observing a vegetarian diet and eating only what is necessary to healthfully sustain our bodies.

Eating a meal can be understood as a *puja,* an act of worship. The Divine comes to the table in the form of food to sustain our lives and to provide us with the energy to serve others. An important *sloka* from the *Bhagavad Gita,* often recited as a meal prayer, states: "The offering is *Brahman* [the Absolute One]. The oblation is *Brahman*, which is offered by *Brahman* into the fire of *Brahman*. The one who sees nothing but *Brahman* in all that he does certainly realizes *Brahman*."

The meal prayer recited daily at Satchidananda Ashram, composed by the great sage Adi Shankaracharya, begins as follows: "Beloved Mother Nature, you are here on our table as our food. You are endlessly bountiful, benefactress of all. Please grant us health and strength, wisdom and dispassion, to find permanent peace and joy, and to share this peace and joy with one and all." Beginning our meal with a prayer can help us to remember this higher purpose and to receive the food with gratitude.

Sri Gurudev explained that, when food is received as a divine offering, it can even bypass the digestive system and be transmuted directly into energy. It is experienced as *prasad*, or a divine blessing. Many years ago, I served as the kitchen mother for our annual retreat in California. We were blessed on the retreat by the presence of Sri Gurudev's longtime devotee, Sohini Mehta. The last meal was a big Indian feast, which I had the opportunity to serve to Sri Gurudev, who was joined at the table by Sohini. As I placed the food on his plate, he would ladle some of it onto hers. Then, when I went to serve Sohini, she immediately placed a big spoonful of the food Gurudev had placed onto her plate directly into my mouth. It felt like sheer electricity. It seemed to explode throughout my system, going everywhere and lighting me from within. The food was not only blessed by him, but doubly blessed by the devotion of this great devotee, and I was the fortunate recipient.

Sri Gurudev spoke about the "3 Ts": the tongue, the time, and the tummy. He cautioned against eating just to satisfy the tongue. There is no end to fulfilling desire in that way, and we are likely to overload our systems with toxins. Likewise, he said not to eat simply because it is mealtime. Instead, check in with your tummy and see if you are hungry. If the hunger is there, you will digest and assimilate the food well. The *Tirukkural* asserts, "There is no need of medicine for the body, if you eat only after making sure that the food already eaten has been digested." Once digestion is complete, eat with moderation. That is the way to prolong the life of the body. The *Bhagavad Gita* gives this assurance, "If you are moderate in eating, playing, sleeping, staying awake, and avoiding extremes in everything you do, you will see these Yoga practices eliminate all your pain and suffering."

Anything we wish to accomplish requires energy. Food provides energy for life—for growth, exploration, and discovery. The way we perform this fundamental, daily act common to all living things, reflects our values, our culture, and our consciousness. By partaking in the proper spirit, we go a long way toward maintaining our health, living in harmony with nature's law, and proving ourselves to be good guardians of our planet's resources.

Really Living Yoga

When I think of what it means to really *live* Yoga, I recall a special visit in late December, in the mid-1970s. I was serving as director of the San Francisco Integral Yoga Institute, and Swami Satchidananda was coming to California for the celebration of his *jayanti* (birthday) in San Francisco, and then he would be with us for Christmas and our New Years retreat in Santa Barbara. It registered hardly more than a week on the calendar, but in the intense whirlwind of love and service that was generated, lessons for a lifetime were learned. These lessons can be understood as basic principles for *really living* Yoga.

The staff at the San Francisco IYI was responsible for coordinating all these events, as well as for housing and hosting the many guests who were coming from all over the country for the festivities. Our very modest living spaces had to be modified and shared in new ways. What at first seemed impossible yielded to our persistent and prayerful efforts. The very walls of the house seemed to expand to accommodate all our guests and the hundreds of students who came to receive Sri Gurudev's blessings. We were few in number, and the task seemed monumental. But by some miracle, everything was accomplished, which brings us to the first principle:

Principle #1: As Sri Gurudev often remarked, "Where there's a will, there's a way. Where there's heart, there's always room."

The weekend began auspiciously. In the morning at the Institute, we had a beautiful *puja* in honor of Sri Gurudev's *jayanti*. In the evening, we enjoyed a wonderful program of offerings at a lovely auditorium in the city. The grand finale was an extraordinary slide show in honor of Sri Gurudev's service. It was so inspiring that, at its conclusion, the entire audience of about seven hundred people jumped to their feet in a standing ovation. This spirit of jubilation continued as some of us proceeded to an Indian restaurant for a late night banquet.

By the time we had finished the meal, it was nearly two in the morning. Gurudev entered an elevator in order to exit the building, and then began calling others to come into the elevator as well. There was a large sign posted inside that read: "Maximum capacity 12 people; do not exceed." With a distinct air of mischief, he beckoned at least twenty of us into that tiny conveyance. When we were all closely crammed in, Gurudev reached forward and pushed the button. The door closed, the elevator started to move, and, then, with a sudden lurch, stopped between floors.

So, there we were in the wee hours of a Sunday morning, trapped in an elevator with our beloved Gurudev. There were devotees on the floors above and below us, chanting and praying. Others began calling all over the city trying to locate a repairman. At this point, I had the thought: "We don't know how long we may be in here. The most important thing is to conserve oxygen. We should all be as still as possible." As if in response to my thought, Gurudev immediately suggested that everyone start chanting *Rama, Rama*—which is a powerful mantra that kindles the inner fire. So, not only would we be using up the physical oxygen, but on a subtle level, we would be creating a lot of heat, too!

As the minutes passed, people began responding in different ways. Some repeatedly tried pushing the buttons. One person tried to climb out the top of the compartment. Some were calm; others panicked. After about forty minutes, Gurudev gently reached over and pressed the button. The elevator immediately proceeded to the ground level, and we all took a deep, grateful breath as we left the building.

On the way back to the Institute, we were discussing what we had just experienced. Finally, the conclusion was that we were being tested to see how we would respond under trying circumstances, and when the test was over, the elevator resumed working. From this experience, we can glean two more principles:

Principle #2: Realize that there is a purpose behind all that unfolds and have faith in a positive outcome.

Principle #3: When faced with challenging circumstances, know that the moment the karma is purged, the situation will change.

As one of my fellow monks has put it: "If it's your karma to have a certain illness, it doesn't matter if you drink nectar, the illness will persist. However, when the karma is drawing to a close, you could even eat dirt, and you would be cured."

The most important lesson of the weekend for me was yet to come. Gurudev was flying down to Santa Barbara, so we all went to see him off at the airport—well, almost all of us. I noticed that one family that had traveled a great distance to be with Gurudev was not present. Upon returning to the Institute, I found them sitting at the reception desk, greeting students coming for the Hatha Yoga class. They innocently asked when they would be able to see Gurudev, not realizing that we all had just come from the airport. It seems that the scheduled receptionist had asked them to reception in her place, so she could go to the airport herself.

It was clear that this was not a good situation and, as the person in charge, I was going to be held accountable. I sensed that trouble lay ahead, but there was so much to do, I couldn't really think about it. So, we all piled into our vehicles, formed a caravan, and proceeded to Santa Barbara. The following evening, we celebrated Christmas with Gurudev and the members from all the California IYIs—from San Francisco, Santa Cruz, Los Angeles, and San Diego. After an inspirational movie, I was making announcements about the retreat that was to begin the following day, when I noticed the guest who had been left behind approach Gurudev. As the guest was speaking, Gurudev kept turning and glancing in my direction. It seemed like each time, there was a little more fire in his eyes.

Then suddenly, Gurudev turned to me and spoke: "All your Yoga practices—your Hatha Yoga, *pranayama*, and meditation are for this purpose: to make you fit to serve others. If ever the opportunity comes to serve, forget those other practices; you can always do them later. Take care of others; that is the most important thing." His words were deeply impressed on my heart. The following day, I offered my apologies, which Gurudev graciously accepted. A couple of essential lessons were learned:

Principle #4: On life's journey, we all make mistakes. However great our capacity to err, the power of forgiveness is greater still. As we would wish to be forgiven, we should practice forgiveness toward one another.

Principle #5: Love all, serve all.

This last one, perhaps, is the greatest of all. It was the message of Gurudev's life. He often quoted the following verse from the *Bhagavad Gita*: "*Tyagat shantir anantaram,*" which means: "The dedicated ever enjoy supreme peace." And he would add, "Therefore, live only to serve."

He compared formal practice and service to a barber giving a shave. Meditation is like sharpening the razor, and service is like shaving. If you don't sharpen the razor, you can't shave well and may even cause harm. If you just spend your time sharpening the razor and don't shave, what is the point?

This blend of the contemplative and active life was the basis for the way he designed the *ashram* schedule, as well as the Integral Yoga retreats, and the way he guided students everywhere to bring Yoga into their lives. By beginning the day with formal practice—meditation and Hatha Yoga—we would condition our minds to stay peaceful and our bodies easeful. Additionally, we could have check-in times throughout the day—at noon, dusk, and before retiring—to center ourselves through prayer and meditation. By so doing, we would be fit for service, and our lives would be useful.

He called each and every one of us to dedicate our lives for the sake of the entire creation: "With every minute, every breath, every atom of our bodies, we should repeat this mantra: dedication, dedication, giving, giving, loving, loving. That is the best Yoga, which will bring us permanent peace and joy." If we do our best to answer this call, then we will really be living Yoga.

TRANSFORMATION

Shifting Our Attitudes and Actions

Swami Satchidananda used to say, "Do your best and leave the rest." That's a good formula for inner transformation.

Transformation is a mysterious process: the caterpillar spins a cocoon and emerges as a butterfly. We can observe the diligent efforts of the caterpillar as it spins the cocoon, but what happens inside remains hidden from view. When we see the beautiful winged creature fly free of its encasement, we know that an intricate, subtle, and delicate series of events has occurred.

Spiritual transformation is similar. We can apply a lot of effort, but the actual transformation occurs beneath the veil of conscious awareness. It's similar to boiling water. We add a lot of energy in the form of heat. We can observe the water getting hotter until it reaches 212 degrees Fahrenheit, but then, something subtle, beyond our perception, occurs. We keep adding heat, but the temperature remains the same. On the spiritual path, this is the point when people sometimes lose heart and give up. Despite all their efforts, they don't see any progress being made. But just as the water finally escapes as steam, the transformation that is happening within eventually becomes visible. Our quantitative efforts result in a qualitative shift.

When we set an intention, we plant a seed that grows within the deeper levels of the mind. With every prayer we utter, we attract divine blessings to back our efforts. Every step we take to change a pattern in our thinking or behavior invests more energy into the process. At a certain point, all these factors converge and we emerge transformed— there's a noticeable shift in our attitudes and actions.

It all begins with a single thought: I want this pattern to change. There's a well-known saying: We sow a thought and reap an action. We repeat an action and it becomes a habit. The sum total of our habits defines our character. And our character, in turn, determines our destiny.

We are the architects of our destiny, more powerful than we realize. The *Yoga Sutras* state that when we persevere for a long time, without break, and in all earnestness, our practice becomes firmly established. At a certain point, within the crucible of our efforts, the most profound transformation occurs—a quintessential change in our state of consciousness. Like the butterfly, we break free of all limitations and soar free in the light.

One Thought at a Time

On this tiny, fragile ball called Earth, we share a common journey. Every day, together, we spin through the vastness of space. Suspended amid the stars, we are born, we grow, and we strive. We have our times of gladness and celebration, and occasions of sorrow and loss. Events don't always unfold in the way we would like; life doesn't always match our picture of how things should be. John Lennon, in one of his songs, noted that, "Life is what happens to you while you're busy making other plans."

There is constant movement, constant change, beginning with our cosmic journey and continuing through the details of our daily existence. No one, no thing, is with us always; nothing remains the same. So it is challenging to keep our peace at all times. In times of hardship or crisis, Swami Satchidananda would often quote an ancient Indian scripture, which proclaims that: "Not even an atom moves without God's will." Nothing can happen without God's permission.

Devoted souls through time eternal have bowed in prayer, uttering: "Thy will be done," affirming total faith, acceptance, and surrender to the higher will. If we have total faith, nothing that happens in life will disturb our peace. We will accept everything as coming from the Higher Power for our highest good. A saintly woman once observed that everyone's life was like a piece of embroidery in which God was fashioning a masterpiece. Most people only viewed it from the backside, and all they saw was a tangle of knotted threads with little meaning. From the proper angle of vision, however, one could see the beauty and purpose that was being fashioned.

So what do we do when life seems harsh, cruel, or pointless; when we are stretched or tested beyond any reasonable limit? How do we respond when our minds are outraged, our hearts bereft of consolation, our bodies broken, and as much as we may want to, we can't truly say, "Not my will, but Thy will be done"? What recourse do we have then? How do we reconcile an all-knowing, all-loving, all-merciful, all-powerful God with all the violence and suffering in the world? Is there a way to understand the workings of God's will so that we can come to peace with what unfolds in life?

In the *Yoga Sutras of Sri Patanjali*, we find a key to unlock this mystery. Patanjali speaks of two eternal principles: *Purusha* (Spirit) and *Prakriti* (nature). *Purusha*, also referred to as the *Atman*, Seer, or Self, is consciousness, the Divine Spirit. *Prakriti* is everything else: the entire creation. Spirit expresses itself through nature. Accordingly, God's will is expressed through the fundamental law of nature, which is the law of karma.

The law of karma, according to Swami Sivananda, states that for every action, there must be a reaction of equal force and similar in nature. The entire universe, comprising everything on the physical and mental planes, unfolds in an orderly way based on this grand law of causation. There is a clear pattern of cause and effect. Sometimes we can readily see the connection: we overeat and get a stomachache. Sometimes the antecedent cause is hidden in the far past.

One thing is certain: If we do good deeds and bring happiness to others, we will experience happiness. If we do harmful acts, harm will come to us. There is no one to blame. As the great South Indian saint, Avvaiyar, once said, "The pleasure and pain we experience in life is not given to us by someone else; we, ourselves, are the cause." Sometime, somewhere, we did something to merit what unfolds in our life. With this understanding, we accept responsibility for our actions and their consequences. Instead of lamenting or protesting about God's will, we take the approach, "My will created this, so my will can change it."

Karma begins with the thoughts we cherish. We sow a thought and reap an action. We repeat an action and it becomes a habit. The sum total of our habits defines our character, and our character, in turn, determines our destiny. This means that everything we are experiencing in our lives—our health or illness, wealth or poverty, happiness or despair—are all due to thoughts we chose to cherish. Every moment is like a slate on which we write our destiny. The destiny we see unfolding in our lives now is none other than the result of thoughts and efforts made in the past, and what we do now will determine the future. We are far more powerful than we realize.

There are three types of karma: *sanchita*, *prarabdha*, and *kriyamana* (also called *agami*). A classical analogy compares karma to an archer with arrows in three stages. There is the quiver filled with arrows, one that has just been released, and another poised in the bow. The quiver represents the *sanchita* karma, the storehouse of all our past actions. All the experiences from previous births remain in the form of impressions, known as *samskaras*, in the subconscious mind. Everything is recorded and retained. The arrow that has been released represents the *prarabdha* karma. This is the inevitable karma, that portion of our karma that has to be worked out in this lifetime. It is like a debt that has come due and cannot be avoided. Then, there is the arrow poised in the bow, which we can choose to release or not. This is the *kriyamana* or *agami*, the new karma we are creating. Here is where our free will can be exercised within certain limitations.

Sri Gurudev compared the scope of free will to a dog tied to a rope of set length. The dog has the freedom to move within the circle defined by the length of the rope. Within that circle, the dog can choose to jump around and bark, dig for bones, or simply lie down and sleep. But the dog cannot accomplish anything outside that circle.

Swami Sivananda describes it this way: Every soul is like a farmer given a plot of land. The acreage, nature of the soil, and weather conditions are all pre-determined (*prarabdha*), but the farmer is at liberty to till, fertilize, and plant to get a good crop or to let the land lie fallow and become wasteland (*agami*).

The law of karma is not fatalistic. Properly understood, it is the ultimate doctrine of self-empowerment. If by our own thoughts and actions we created a situation, then it is within our power to create another more to our liking. This takes patience and perseverance. The *Tirukkural*, a holy scripture from South India, states: "One should never get disheartened thinking a job is difficult of execution; perseverance will give you the capacity to do it."

More importantly, karma can be transcended altogether. The *sanchita* and *agami* will eventually be destroyed when one attains God-realization. The *prarabdha* must be experienced but, with divine grace and a proper attitude, we can deal with it skillfully. According to the Jewish tradition, on the first day of the New Year, one's fate is inscribed and, on the tenth day, it is sealed. In the interim, through prayer, penance, and charity, severe decrees can be averted. In like manner, a South Indian proverb declares, "For a devotee of God, an arrow that comes for the head, takes the hat instead." Thus, through faith, prayer, atonement, and good deeds, karma can be mitigated.

There is an Islamic saying: "Trust in God, but tie up your camel." In other words, don't worry, have faith in God; and at the same time, do all that you can to move things along in a positive direction. This is true in our personal lives and with respect to the world as well. The news today is filled with stories of conflicts and problems, of disasters—both natural and man-made. Just as our individual thoughts have determined our personal circumstances, so, too, our cumulative collective consciousness has produced the world, as we know it. There is individual karma, national karma, and even global karma. Our lives and our destinies are intertwined.

In the mid-1970s in California, there were many natural disasters, including fire, flood, and earthquake. We had an *ashram* in Santa Barbara, and many of our family members had homes in the next town, Montecito, where a big fire occurred. Our members' homes were located right in the path of the fire, so they fled to the *ashram* for refuge. As we listened to reports of the blaze, we were struck by the comments: "This fire seems to have a mind of its own. It goes in one direction, burns a house; then, for no apparent reason, makes a turn, skips two houses, and burns another." There was no apparent logic to what they were observing. When the fire was finally extinguished, our members returned, intending to rake the rubble in search of valuables, only to find that every one of their homes had been spared.

Similarly, there was flooding in southern California, with reports of the ocean seeming to consciously engulf particular houses and draw them back in to itself. We asked Sri Gurudev what was going on, and he responded that, "There is consciousness everywhere. The very elements respond to our thoughts. If nature is abused or misused, you will see a response of this sort."

Here is the good news: If we had a share in creating the events that we see unfolding, we also have the power to positively impact them as well. A major earthquake in California was predicted by many people—including scientists, religious leaders, and astrologers—but it never occurred. When asked to comment, Sri Gurudev replied that it was because of all the people who were praying.

We are all guardians of this planet, entrusted with a small, but essential, role to play. The Reverend Martin Luther King, Jr. once said, "We are caught in an inescapable network of mutuality, tied in a single garment of destiny. Whatever affects one directly, affects all indirectly." We may not be in a position to set government policy or influence the practices of major corporations, but by our own thoughts and efforts, we contribute in a very real way to how events unfold.

Swami Sivananda wrote: "Every thought that you send out is a vibration which never perishes. It goes on vibrating every particle of the universe and if your thoughts are noble, holy and forcible, they set in vibration every sympathetic mind. Unconsciously, all people who are like you take the thought you have projected and in accordance with the capacity that they have, they send out similar thoughts. The result is that, without your knowledge of the consequences of your own work, you will be setting in motion great forces which will work together and put down the lowly and mean thoughts generated by the selfish and the wicked."

So let us begin where we are and carry this positive spirit into our family, workplace, school, and community. We can change our destiny and we can change the world, one thought at a time.

Strategies for Transformation

Everywhere in nature, we see change. Day gives way to night. The hot and humid days of summer yield to the brisk, cool winds of fall. The garden is in bloom, and then goes to seed. Similarly, the circumstances in our own lives are always in flux.

We live in an ocean of change. We are a microcosm of the universe. The same laws that we see in the macrocosm are operative in us as well. Then, why do we sometimes feel powerless to make changes in our lives? Why do we get stuck in undesirable habits or situations? Why do some obstacles seem insurmountable, certain problems unsolvable? It seems like a paradox.

Very often the answer is quite simple: we don't make changes because we don't believe we can. The *Yoga Sutras of Patanjali* lists doubt as one of the main obstacles on the spiritual path. Even a little doubt can undermine everything. It's like putting a thimbleful of poison into a pot of nectar; the entire pot will be tainted. Or like a grain of sand falling into a large, complex machine; the whole mechanism will come grinding to a halt. Wallace Black Elk, a Native American teacher and spiritual leader, once shared stories of healings he had witnessed. He said that Mother Nature was always ready to heal us; what stood in the way was our doubt.

Change is always possible. Swami Satchidananda was a master in the art of transformation. A moment in his presence could change a life completely. The glance of a spiritual master is said to be like a raft that can carry one across the ocean of *samsara*, this turbulent sea of comings and goings, ups and downs. The power of grace can also flow through a simple act of loving-kindness by a friend. Even if our confidence in ourselves is shaky, the timely and caring support of another can make what may seem impossible, doable. The gift of love is a potent force for growth, renewal, and change.

Transformation can also be the fruit of self-effort. The teachings of Integral Yoga include techniques that are powerful tools for making changes in our lives. They utilize the will, the heart, or the intellect, corresponding to the different aspects of an individual. When applied with faith and determination, these strategies provide a roadmap that can help us reach our goals.

Applying the Will

The first approach involves application of the will. The *Tirukkural* states, "There is nothing that is impossible if one brings to bear on one's work the instrument of a vigilant and resourceful mind." The will can be applied in any area of life with success. We see this, not only with respect to spiritual endeavor, but also in the sports arena, in political campaigns, in scientific research, and in business pursuits— wherever there is a contest of strength, a new discovery in the making, or focused effort to attain a chosen objective.

Michael Jordan once said, "I visualized where I wanted to be, what kind of player I wanted to become. I knew exactly where I wanted to go, and I focused on getting there." About obstacles along the way, he said, "If you're trying to achieve, there will be roadblocks. I've had them. Everybody has had them, but obstacles don't have to stop you. If you run into a wall, don't turn around and give up. Figure out how to climb it, go through it, or work around it."

Great inventors have the same kind of determination. Thomas Edison experimented with over 10,000 prototypes before he came up with a viable light bulb. About this process, he commented: "I have not failed 10,000 times. I have not failed once. I have succeeded in proving that those 10,000 ways will not work. When I have eliminated the ways that will not work, I will find the way that will work."

You, too, can activate the will to accomplish your goals and effect positive change in your life. The first step is simply to have the willingness, the desire, to make a change. Next, define your goal, set an intention of what you wish to achieve. An infinite ocean of cosmic energy surrounds us. Intention aligns us to receive and direct that power in a particular way. Setting an intention is like planting a seed in the mind. Quietly, in the background, the seed sprouts and draws to it the resources needed for its growth. Sri Gurudev used to say that the entire cosmos is there to bless our efforts, silently intoning, "*Tathastu*," which means, "Be it so."

It's often helpful to divide the task into doable steps. It's unrealistic to expect longstanding patterns or situations to change overnight. Using the will is like building a muscle: Apply weights that challenge, but don't overwhelm it. That way the mind will grow in confidence and strength. Finally, focus your mind on the task. Make a *sankalpa*, a strong resolve that you will attain your goal. Sri Gurudev used to say that if you make a *sankalpa*, "Every cell, every atom, of your being will hear and obey. They are waiting for you to reassert your mastery." If your mind 100 percent wants to do something, you will be successful.

Turning to Prayer

Sometimes even though we apply our will, our strength proves unequal to the task. At such times, one can always turn to prayer. Once I was dealing with a big obstacle. Sri Gurudev met with me and told me to use my will to overcome it. I spent the next year doing everything I could to tackle that obstacle: I tried going over it, under it, and around it, but all my efforts proved futile. At the end of that period, Sri Gurudev asked to speak with me again. He gently inquired, "So, how has it been going with using your will?" A year's worth of frustration poured forth as I replied, "Going? It hasn't gone anywhere. Nothing has changed." Then, he laughed and said, "So, now we see what your will can accomplish in this situation. There is only one thing left to do. Just throw your hands in the air and cry to God."

At other times, even though we know we should make a change, we don't seem to have the will to do so. In such cases, we can begin by praying for the desire to make the change. Once the desire is there, pray for guidance. When you receive the guidance, pray for strength. When the desire, guidance, and strength all converge, then make your move. You may be surprised to see that what seemed like an immovable boulder blocking your path, will gently crumble like fine powder.

Sincere prayer is always answered. When we call out with our whole heart, the help comes. The Higher Power is always there to back our efforts. We are like gadgets that can operate either on battery or plug-in. If we run on battery power, we have limited capacity. If we plug in, we can draw unlimited energy. We seem to have forgotten that there is a universal outlet, and that we can connect and draw all the support that we need.

One morning many years ago, when I was living at our *ashram* in Santa Barbara, I awoke in great despair, feeling that I would never attain my spiritual goal. I called Gurudev and told him that all I wanted was to realize God, but I didn't feel I had the capacity. There was silence on the other end of the phone, and then I heard, "click."

I couldn't believe it; he hung up on me! I had expected some words of encouragement or reassurance. Instead, I got "click." I concluded that not only were my fears justified, but rather than confirm them, Sri Gurudev chose, out of compassion, to say nothing.

That evening we had *satsang*. Normally, Sri Gurudev would go directly to answering questions. That evening, he simply gazed around the room. When he caught my eye, he said, "Some of you might feel you don't have the strength to realize the higher truth, that it is beyond your capacity. You are right! But you don't have to do it alone. The Higher Power is always there to help you. And with that backing, anything is possible!"

Shining the Light of Awareness

Another approach is simply shining the light of awareness on the problem. Observation alone will cause a shift to happen without any further effort. Even in science, the Heisenberg Uncertainty Principle states that the mere presence of an observer in an experiment causes changes to occur. We all know that we behave differently if someone is watching us.

Recently, I was at a computer store, when in walked a man who was obviously very frustrated about an issue with his device that had not been resolved. As he became increasingly angry, the staff went on alert and summoned the mall security officer. The officer simply stood to the side and watched the interaction. He never said a word or did anything. He just observed and, by his mere presence, everything shifted and the man calmed down. Similarly, when we move into a witnessing mode, our undesirable mental and behavioral patterns are exposed and become less likely to express themselves.

When we step back and observe, it's like turning off a main switch. It's our involvement that energizes our behaviors. This separation immediately divests them of energy. When you can watch something, it's clear that the thing in question is not you. You see it more objectively and can understand it more clearly. This distance between the observer and the observed provides a window in which you can choose whether to pursue or change your course.

This technique can be practiced along with introspection. First, identify the behavior you wish to change. Then, every evening, replay the tape of your day, making special note of when that pattern occurred. Don't judge, just observe. If self-judgment or criticism slips into the exercise, the process will be compromised. The mind's defenses will be triggered and its armor raised, blocking the penetrating light.

After practicing regularly for some time, when you re-play the tape at night, you will begin to notice the factors that precipitate the pattern you are trying to change. You will be able to clearly observe the whole episode: the precursors, your reaction, and the ensuing consequences. This expanded awareness will slowly begin to percolate into your daily life, so that as the event unfolds, you will be aware of every aspect.

Then, when you do your nightly introspection, you will be able to see not only the event, but also the presence of your awareness as it unfolded. Gradually, that awareness will open up a space within you in which time seems to slow down. Instead of being caught in habitual, automatic, and reactive patterns, you will have the opportunity to establish new ones.

I used this technique while working with anger. Anger is a powerful force, difficult to overcome directly. So, I tried this indirect approach. After practicing regularly for some time, I discovered the inner workings of this technique as described above. For many months, the anger persisted because of past momentum. But slowly, the option of choice began to enter. And on one fine day, I finally chose not to get angry. The sense of freedom was wonderful.

Positive transformation is always possible. You may encounter setbacks, but if you keep at it, success will be yours. Never give up. Never lose hope. Use your will, turn to prayer, shine the light of awareness. And when you feel the winds of grace blowing, open your sails and catch the breeze. Peace, happiness, and freedom await you.

As You Think, So You Become

There is a Sanskrit saying often quoted by Swami Satchidananda: "*Mana eva manushyanam karanam bandha mokshayoh.*" It means: "As the mind, so the individual. Bondage or liberation is in the mind." In other words, As you think, so you become. If you think well, you become well; if you think ill, you will become ill. The mind is that powerful.

There is a story that beautifully illustrates this principle. It is about the man whose words are quoted on the Shinto altar in the Light Of Truth Universal Shrine (LOTUS) at Yogaville. His name was Kurozumi Munetada, and he lived in the 19th century in Japan.

When he was a young man, his parents suddenly died, one after another. He was plunged into such profound and prolonged sorrow that he became very ill himself. Negative emotions are known to affect particular organs in the body. Sorrow goes to the lungs, and he developed consumption of the lungs.

His condition worsened, until one day the doctor came to visit and told him that he had little time left, that there was nothing more that could be done for him. Kurozumi lay on his deathbed and began to reflect: "Have I honored the memory of my beloved parents by grieving so much that now I, too, am at the point of death? Probably, they are looking down upon me and are filled with so much sadness to see my condition." Then and there, he resolved to put aside all grieving and embrace instead the spirit of gratefulness, giving thanks for all the blessings in his life. He didn't know if it would change his fate, but thought that, at least, it might bring some comfort to the spirits of his departed parents.

Kurozumi wished to gaze upon the sun one more time, because in Japan, the sun represents Amaterasu O-mi-kami, the Sun Goddess. In his weakened condition, with a heart full of gratitude, he prayed intensely to the Goddess. As the rays of the sun penetrated him, he experienced a mystical union with the Goddess and had a profound spiritual awakening. His physical health was restored and he was blessed with the power to heal others. Following that experience, he founded a new sect of the Shinto faith, called the Kurozumi sect.

Sri Patanjali, in the *Yoga Sutras*, presents the technique of *pratipaksha bhavana*, replacing a negative thought with an opposite positive one. Kurozumi Munetada probably never read the *Yoga Sutras*, but he implemented one of its principles with dramatic results. Negative thinking had brought him to death's door; positive thinking resulted in physical and mental well-being, as well as spiritual awakening. We, too, can turn to this practice and triumph over negative attitudes, habits or situations in our lives. We are more powerful than we realize.

Walk with Faith

Once a group of scientists had a meeting and decided that they no longer needed God— that they could do everything God could do by themselves. So, they selected a representative to tell God of their decision. God graciously granted an interview. After the scientist had conveyed the wishes of his group, God said that was fine. But after a moment, with a twinkle in the eye, God asked, "Would you like to have a contest?" The scientist said, "Sure." And God said, "How about a man-making contest?" And the scientist said, "Okay, we know how to do that now." And God said, "Let's do it the way I did it in the beginning, from the earth itself." The man replied, "All right; we have even figured out how to do that." So, God said, "Great. Let's do it: ready, set, go!" The man reached down to scoop up a handful of earth. And God said, "No, no, no. Go get your own earth."

In our arrogance and our ignorance, our confusion and fear, we forget that Higher Power that has set billions of galaxies in place within the fabric of the universe and has ordered their movements through time and space. We overlook the incomparable artistry and tenderness that could create a flower—one with the intricacy of an orchid, the fragrance of jasmine, or the beauty of a single red rose. We become enamored of our fleeting achievements, attached to the tiny bundle of possessions we manage to amass. We forget the awesome splendor of this world in which we dwell. We forget the great hand, the great heart, that created it and placed each one of us here with a purpose to fulfill.

So, here we are: Seven billion people, along with countless numbers and varieties of vegetation and creatures, all spinning through space on this tiny ball we call Earth. By some miracle, we don't fall off. With each turn, we mark a day. With each revolution around the sun, we add a year to our lives. Amid the whirling and twirling, we have our successes and failures, our triumphs and tragedies. Albert Einstein once said, "There are two ways to live your life. One is as though nothing is a miracle. The other is as though everything is a miracle."

When we see the manifest universe, we are witnessing an extraordinary creation, an effect as it were. Whenever we see an effect, there must be a prior cause. So, seeing the creation, we can infer the existence of a Creator. And that is where faith comes in. St. Augustine said, "Faith is to believe what we do not see, and the reward of this faith is to see what we believe."

Believing without seeing: How can this be done? We often say, "Seeing is believing." But if we reflect for a moment, there are numerous examples in life of the power of the invisible. Take electricity for example. We don't see it, but we infer its existence from all the devices that we see powered by it. In the practice of homeopathy, the higher the potency of a remedy, the less actual medicinal substance is present. In the really powerful remedies, there is not even a single physical molecule of the medicinal substance—only its subtle, vibrational pattern. If you compare an atom to a bullet with respect to the destruction it can render, it's clear that the atom, which is invisible, is the more powerful of the two.

To explore this a little further, anything that is constant in our perceptual field becomes invisible to us. The mind and senses are set up to detect change. How many people hear the constant hum of their refrigerator? A guest entering might find it disturbing at first; but after a while, it blends into the background. We are whirling through space at tremendous speed—does anyone feel the movement?

What we call God is the supreme constant in the universe, and as such, is invisible to our physical senses. It is the stable, unchanging support of the entire creation. If we go to a movie theater, the screen is stable and unchanging. If not for the screen, we couldn't even see the film. But in general, we never notice the screen, just the passing images. So, too, we don't perceive God, only the diverse names and forms. The fact that we're perceiving all the changes is proof that there must be something unchanging behind them—just like we wouldn't be able to see a multi-colored painting, unless there were a neutral canvas behind it. From this perspective, experiencing God could be described as a fundamental shift, in which the stable support becomes prominent in our awareness, instead of the changing phenomena.

I once had a glimpse of what this would be like when I was living at our *ashram* in Santa Barbara. One morning, it was my task to take one of the cars to the repair shop to be serviced. I was not very happy about doing this because it necessitated cutting my practices short and going to a part of town that I didn't particularly like. So, I drove downtown and left the car with the mechanic. It was early, and traffic was heavy as people rushed to work. All the shops were still closed, so I decided to take a walk. And then, all of a sudden, everything changed. Where one moment before, all had been hustle and bustle, now there was only peace—pure, perfect, complete peace—everywhere. It was as if the background of peace that is always there came forward. The traffic and all the commotion receded into the background.

Until such time as we perceive that perfect peace continually, we can cultivate and reaffirm our faith in that which we cannot see. We often say: "Good things come in small packages." The best come in invisible ones.

How can we do that? How can we have faith in the invisible? Every single day we are taught the lesson of faith. We say the darkest hour is before the dawn. Just imagine: It's been dark all night; and now it's getting darker, and darker, and darker still. At that point, a small bird leaps onto a branch and begins to sing with all her heart, because she knows the big red ball is going to rise in the sky. That is faith. Rabindranath Tagore, the great poet of India, said, "Faith is the bird that feels the light and sings when the dawn is still dark."

Very often it is in our darkest hours that we learn to walk with faith. When we are presented with problems beyond our capacity to solve, with situations beyond our ability to understand, we turn to a Higher Power, a higher wisdom, for guidance and light. At such times, a person of faith would believe as St. Paul did, "All things work for the good for those who love God." He would trust that there is an ultimate, benevolent purpose behind all that transpires and that adversities are blessings in disguise. This is the test of faith: the degree to which our will is at one with the higher will.

The highest faith is total acceptance, total surrender to the higher will. This is not easy to do. But this was the way of all the saints. If you look at the lives of the saints from any of the world's faiths, the measure of their sanctity was their faith and ability to surrender to the higher will. Here are some striking examples.

One of my favorites is St. Teresa of Avila. On many occasions, Jesus would come and speak to her directly. Once he commanded her to open another convent. She immediately made preparations, and on the next day was ready to depart. A friend stopped her and questioned where she was going. Teresa told her that she had received a divine command to start another convent. Her friend remarked, "Teresa, you only have five *ducats* in your pocket. How are you going to make the journey, purchase the building, establish the convent, and then make the return trip home?"

Teresa thought a moment before responding: "You are right. Teresa and five *ducats* can do nothing. But God, Teresa, and five *ducats* can do anything!" She went, and it was accomplished.

In the *Holy Bible*, Jesus says, "If you have faith the size of a mustard seed, you shall say to the mountain 'come hither' and it will come; and nothing will be impossible to you." How much faith did he say was needed? A mustard seed. Probably, he picked that as an example because it was the smallest thing people were familiar with on a daily basis. He didn't say a basketful, or a cartload, or a barn full of faith; he chose the smallest thing around.

Another saintly personality, from the Islamic faith, was Rabi'a al-'Adawiyya, who lived in the 8th century. Once Rabi'a was seen running with fire in one hand and water in the other. When asked what she was doing, she replied that she was going to set fire to heaven and put out the fire in hell, so that both veils would disappear for true pilgrims. Then they would seek God not out of fear of hell nor desire for heaven, but only for the love of God.

During an illness, Rabi'a was once visited by two pious friends. One of them suggested that she pray to God to relieve her suffering.

In gentle reproof, she reminded him that it was God who willed her suffering. And she added, "Why do you bid me ask for what is contrary to His will? It is not well to oppose one's Beloved."

In the Jewish tradition, there is the story of Rabbi Zushe, who was very poor and endured many hardships in life. Nevertheless, he was always happy. He studied under the holy Magid of Mezeritch. One day, some of the rabbinical students were trying to understand a passage in the *Talmud* about blessing the Almighty for misfortune with the same joy as when one blesses the Almighty for good fortune. When they asked their holy teacher for an explanation, the Magid told them to go and ask Rabbi Zushe. When they put the question to Rabbi Zushe, he seemed surprised that they would ask him such a thing. He then explained, "You had better ask someone who suffered some misfortune in his life. I have never experienced anything bad in my life. Only good things have happened to me." That is true faith and acceptance of God's will. Acceptance does not mean gritting your teeth and bearing with what comes. It means embracing God's will with total joy.

In the Hindu tradition, there is a wonderful example of the power of faith in the life of Draupadi. She was a noble queen who lived in ancient times. In order to disgrace her husbands, she was dragged into the royal court to be disrobed. (She had five husbands—but that's another story!) A strong man came forward and unwrapped one round of her *sari*. She was clutching the *sari* with all her might, at the same time calling out to God in the form of Krishna to save her. But her strength was no match for that of her assailant, and soon another round of the *sari* was undone. There was one more round to go, when a great light dawned within her. She realized she couldn't save herself with her own strength. At that point, she just threw her arms in the air and cried out, "Krishna, save me if you will: my honor, my disgrace are in your hands." She had reached the level of total surrender.

That is when the miracle happened. After the last round, there was another, and another, and still another. Yards and yards of *sari* seemed to be coming from out of nowhere. Finally, the fellow collapsed from exhaustion next to the huge mound of cloth that he had unwrapped, while Draupadi remained fully clothed and protected.

In the Zen tradition, too, there is a story that equates sanctity with this quality of acceptance. It is about the Japanese master Hakuin, who was revered as a pure and holy man. It happened that a young girl in the village became pregnant. When asked by her parents who the father was, she named Hakuin. The angry parents brought the child to him and demanded that he raise it, since he was the father. All he said was, "Is that so?" He accepted and cared for the child. He lost his good name, but that didn't bother him at all.

A year later, the girl confessed that the father of her child was really a young man who worked in the fish market. Again, the parents went to Hakuin and this time implored that he return the child, since he was not the father. And again, all that he said as he gave the child back was, "Is that so?"

Faith, acceptance, and surrender is the way of those who walk with God and walk in peace. For some people, faith comes naturally. But even if it doesn't, there are ways we can develop it. Here are some practical suggestions for deepening faith and cultivating it in daily life:

1. We've all heard the expression: "Seeing the world through rose-colored glasses." Every morning when you get up, imagine that you are putting on faith-colored glasses. Choose to see the world through the eyes of faith. If you seek to see God's hand and grace in all that transpires, you will develop that vision.

2. Every morning, make a list of your plans for the day; every evening, review what actually transpired. You will soon become convinced that a Higher Power is at work in your life.

3. Think about all the benefits and gifts you have received in your life. The more you think of them, the more grateful you will feel, and the more devoted you will become. Brother David Steindl-Rast asserts, "Gratefulness is the heart of prayer."

4. A great physician used to recommend to people with serious illnesses that every day they write down five blessings in their life. At the end of the week, they were to review the entire list. This would help to instill hope and faith, which would, in turn, promote healing.

5. Swami Satchidananda says that, in order to grow in faith, we should cultivate the attitude, "I believe in God. I have given myself into God's hands. Whatever happens does so because God allows it to happen, and it's for my good. If it were not for my good, why would God allow it to happen? Is God not powerful? Am I not God's beloved?" That's what you called true devotion, true faith in God.

6. When you are trying to cultivate faith, there will be tests. When tests come, pray sincerely. You will receive all the strength and guidance you need. By facing difficult situations in this way, your faith will deepen.

7. Never get discouraged or give in to despair. When difficulties come, trust in God's mercy and grace, and don't get disheartened by your own limitations. A traditional prayer to the *Bhagavad Gita* states that God's grace "makes the mute eloquent and the crippled cross mountains." A saintly woman once said, "It is not a great faith that we need, just faith in a great God."

8. Be regular in your meditation and other spiritual practices. Regular *sadhana* will clean the mind, purify the heart, and help you to grow in faith and devotion.

9. Gather together with fellow seekers for support. If you wish to grow in faith, keep company with others who are also cultivating it. You will inspire one another, and together, you will learn how to walk more and more with faith.

No More Fear

One warm summer day, a young man lay down and had a dream in which he traveled the world to broaden his knowledge and seek his fortune. After many years, he came upon a charming village, replete with fertile fields and inhabited by very good and gracious people. There he met a beautiful woman whom he wed. He purchased some farmland and, together, they worked and raised a family.

Many years passed and they prospered. One day, torrential rains began to pour. It rained and rained, and the land became flooded. The harvest was destroyed. The waters rose, and as his house was about to collapse, he quickly gathered up his wife and three children onto their small boat and started rowing. The waters were swirling with tremendous force. The boat was too heavy for him to control; he could scarcely row. He was faced with a terrible dilemma. If things continued much longer, they would all perish. If they were to have any chance of survival, he would have to lighten the load. His mind was reeling with fear and apprehension.

Should he toss the children overboard? His wife? His mind recoiled in horror at the thought. "Perhaps, I can jump overboard," he mused for a moment, and then quickly realized that there would be no one left to row the boat. What should he do?

Actually, there was a very simple solution. He could just wake up! After all, it was only a dream. In the short telling of this tale, how many of you remembered that it was only a dream? Likewise, the Hindu scriptures tell us that life as we know it—this shifting play of names and forms—is a dream of sorts. We are asleep to the truth. Instead of delighting in the peace and perfection of reality, we are continually tossed by the ups and downs inherent in duality.

Waking up is easier said than done. It may all be an illusion, but the pain can feel very real. The mind changes like the weather, and unless and until we attain an enlightened state of awareness, we can find ourselves affected by these shifting conditions. Yoga can help by offering various approaches to enable us to more skillfully deal with unsettling thoughts and feelings when they arise. This is important not only for our mental well-being, but for our physical health as well.

Samuel Hahneman, the founder of homeopathy, stated that the origin of disease is wrong thinking. The mind and body are not simply connected—they are the same stuff at different densities, different rates of vibration. Body is solidified mind. Our body is an expression of the thoughts we have cultivated.

There is a story from the life of Abraham Lincoln that illustrates this principle. He was considering candidates for a position in his cabinet. One person had the right qualifications, but President Lincoln was reluctant to enlist his services. When asked the reason for his hesitation, Lincoln replied, "I don't like his face." When questioned whether that was sufficient reason not to engage the man for a position for which he was qualified, Lincoln explained, "After the age of forty, everyone is responsible for his face!"

The ancient science of Ayurveda tells us that unresolved emotions have a significant role in causing illness. Repressed anger changes the flora of the gallbladder and small intestine. Fear and anxiety alter the flora of the large intestine. Repressed fear affects the kidneys; anger affects the liver; greed affects the heart and the spleen. So we don't want to suppress emotions; that will only cause disease. The yogic key to dealing with disturbing emotions is to redirect the mind through practice and, by so doing, to gain the capacity to release them. Depending on one's temperament, there are four basic approaches that reflect the four basic yogic paths.

If you have an emotional nature, there's the path of devotion known as Bhakti Yoga. When troubled, you can redirect the mind toward the Divine. Instead of focusing on your own limitations, you look with faith and hope to the mercy and grace of God. You can turn to prayer and release your problems into God's tender care. By accepting the higher will, you regain and retain your peace and balance in life.

An intellectual seeker will take a Jnana Yoga approach. This entails observation and analysis. You redirect your attention so that you are no longer identified with the mental disturbance. Stepping back, you become the observer as thoughts and feelings pass through the mind. With this neutral stance comes greater understanding. With understanding comes the capacity for release.

For those who like to use their will, there's the path of Raja Yoga. Through discipline, you purify, strengthen, and harmonize the body, breath, and mind. You withdraw the mind from undesirable thoughts by consciously cultivating positive ones. As two physical objects cannot occupy the same space at the same time, so, too, two contrary thoughts cannot occupy the mind simultaneously. By establishing new habits, you supplant negative patterns.

For those who are action-oriented, there is the path of Karma Yoga. You redirect the mind by engaging in selfless service. By thinking of others more, you dwell on your own problems less. There's a Chinese proverb that says: "If you want to be happy for an hour, take a nap. If you want to be happy for a day, go fishing. If you want to be happy for a month, get married; for a year, inherit a fortune. But if you want to be happy always, serve others."

Swami Satchidananda was once asked to address the medical staff at the University of Virginia Medical Center. He walked up to a blackboard on the stage and wrote two words: Illness and Wellness. Next, he circled the "I" in illness and the "We" in wellness, and then he took his seat. When asked to explain, he said selfishness gives rise to illness, whereas always thinking of the common good and how you can serve others promotes health. A study was once done that showed that the more often a person used the words, "I, me, and mine," the more likely that person was to suffer from heart disease. Evidence has also demonstrated that people who have a good support system tend to recover better compared to those who are isolated and alone.

Dealing with Fear

Most of us deal with fear at some points in our lives. There are real dangers and overwhelming situations that we may have to face. Our whole physiology shifts gears; our glands and nerves get pumped up to enable us to respond in ways beyond our normal capacity. This type of fear can be protective and serve a useful purpose.

Fear becomes problematic when there is no real danger at hand, and it is mostly rooted in imagination and anticipation. Here we often see its common variants, like worry, anxiety, and dread, come into play. These deplete our energy, weaken the immune system, and can destroy the quality of our lives. Most things people are afraid of never come to pass, or not in the way they imagined. A Chinese proverb puts it this way: "Worry is like a blind man, in a dark alley, looking for a black cat that never existed." Real crises usually come unexpected, and, somehow, we find the strength and courage to face them.

I have dealt with fear in my life—one in particular that was longstanding. My teacher, Swami Satchidananda, helped me to understand and overcome it. The first approach was analysis, which revealed that the root of fear is attachment. We don't want to lose something—it could be our health, a possession, a friend, our reputation—or any number of things that are important to us. The first link in this chain of attachment is attachment to our body, to life itself. From there, we become attached to anything we feel we need to support or enhance our lives.

So, the first advice he gave me was to undermine the root cause of all fear, by formulating an affirmation that I was not afraid of death. When I sat for meditation, I was to say the affirmation several times before the period of mantra repetition. The power of the mantra would then go to fulfill the intention behind my affirmation.

Affirmations should be short, clear, and stated in the present tense. If you place your affirmation in the future, that future may always elude you. You can record the affirmation and play it often. That way the message gets instilled into the subconscious mind. Sri Gurudev compared it to an old-fashioned grease job on a car—when you super-inject new grease into the engine, the old grease is ejected. Similarly, when you cultivate new thoughts, the old, undesirable ones are replaced.

Next, as a powerful antidote to fear, Gurudev told me to totally rely on God and to have faith that God was always taking care of me, and that everything happens for our highest good. That was easy to do in theory, but then he told me to repeat the following prayer with all my heart: "God, do whatever you want to me!" That was not so easy to do, because I had the sense that "Someone" was listening and I didn't know what sort of response my prayer would elicit. But I did as he directed and, after some time, the very utterance of the prayer brought a tremendous sense of freedom and connectedness to the Higher Power. It felt like we were on the same team, and so, there was absolutely nothing to fear. As Gurudev often said, "Faith and fear don't go together." If we attach ourselves to God, we can detach from fear.

Gurudev told me to think of fear when it entered the mind like an unwanted guest. If you don't entertain it, it will leave more quickly. Don't probe into it; the more you think about it, the more you encourage it. Instead, starve it like a weed. If it persists, you can talk to or dialogue with it. I tried this at the dentist. For many days, I had been dreading a procedure I was to undergo. Once in the chair, I began talking to the pain. I discovered that if you face your fear, it will dissipate. Fear is like a bully. If you cower before it, it will puff itself up. If you face it, it will shrink to a mere nothing. The actual physical pain was not nearly as bad as the fear of the pain that had preceded it.

Daily *pranayama* (yogic breathing techniques) and meditation were also part of the regimen. *Pranayama* enhances your inner vitality, and prolonged repetition of the mantra surrounds you with a protective vibrational shield. Whenever I did alternate breathing, I employed the *pratipaksha bhavana* technique of Raja Yoga for overcoming a negative pattern. I breathed in faith and courage and exhaled the fear.

After several years, a day came when I had to face the situation again. The best-case scenario that I envisioned was that the fear would rise up, but I would now have the strength to push it aside. Instead, there was no fear at all. Absolutely none! I turned my gaze inward and searched every nook and cranny of my mind, only to find that a longstanding pattern was no longer there. In that moment, I was filled with profound gratitude for Sri Gurudev's wisdom and tender care. I understood, in a new and deeply personal way, the power of the practices and the freedom that comes from self-mastery. That freedom awaits us all, and the practices are a proven means to attain it.

The Gift of Healing

Swami Satchidananda used to say that God laughs on two occasions. The first is when two neighbors erect a fence and declare, "This is mine, and that is yours." The second time is when a patient recovers, and the doctor proudly proclaims, "I cured him."

In the *Yoga Sutras of Patanjali, sutra* 4.3 states: "Incidental events do not directly cause natural evolution; they just remove the obstacles, as a farmer removes the obstacles in a water course running to his field." From the yogic perspective, the physician doesn't cure the patient. Instead, he or she helps remove the impediments, all the toxins and tensions that have built up in the system, so the divine healing energy within the individual can flow unobstructed. A course of treatment is prescribed that will help restore the patient's natural strength and immunity. At the same time, he or she is asked to avoid introducing new toxins into the system or doing anything that could cause harm. From ancient times, we have the medical dictum: "First, do no harm." This is totally in keeping with the yogic approach.

In his youth, Swami Satchidananda prayed for and received the gift of healing. People would come to him with all sorts of problems, and he would heal them. After some time, he began to feel uncomfortable, that he was doing something wrong. He would heal them, but they would continue with the same bad habits that had caused the illness in the first place and, after some time, the problems would recur. So he changed his approach. Instead, he gave them dietary advice, instructed them in yogic techniques, and then silently added his prayers. That way, they corrected their behavior, and the results were lasting. By their own efforts, they purged their karma, and his ego was spared the temptation of taking any credit.

It is important for those pursuing the healing arts to keep any ego out of the mix. Practitioners can offer their skills, techniques, medicines, prayers, and support. They may do all that they can, but the result is not in their hands. Healing is divine. Sometimes the treatment is perfect; an operation is successful, yet the patient doesn't survive. True healing doesn't always mean that the body recovers. Sometimes the body dies, but the patient has healed—learned the necessary lessons, resolved past issues, and come to peace. Death isn't a failure; it is inevitable. And from the yogic perspective, it provides us with an opportunity for a fresh start.

The yogic approach to healing is being sought today by multitudes, who are frustrated by the limitations and undesirable side effects of western medicine. Drawing from ancient wisdom, Yoga has various practices and principles, strategies and techniques, to offer. Beyond all that, yogic practitioners can bring the gift of their own healing vibrations to a therapeutic setting. By living in accordance with the ethical precepts of *yama* and *niyama*, as well as maintaining a regular practice of disciplines to keep the body and mind clean and strong, an energetic charge is developed in the system. This high vibratory field can help to quicken the divine force within others, so healing can occur.

Sri Gurudev used to say that teaching Yoga is not like teaching geography. We are not simply conveying information, rather a little bit of spiritual energy is transmitted as well. We can't give what we don't have, so first we need to develop that energy within ourselves. First we practice; then we share what we've gathered and learned. After some time, all we need do is live, and others will get the benefit from simply being in our presence. It's not that we try to heal others. The sun doesn't try to dispel the darkness. Its nature is to give light; by virtue of its presence, the darkness flees.

There's a Hassidic story about a very good man. One day God spoke to him and offered him a boon. The man humbly replied, "Lord, in your compassion, you have deigned to speak with me. What more could I ask?" But the Lord insisted, so the man thought deeply and finally requested: "Whenever I am departing a town and walking such that my shadow is behind me, let blessings occur wherever my shadow falls." And so it came to pass. In the wake of his shadow, the earth was fruitful, healing occurred, and peace was restored, without any knowledge or conscious action on his part. He came to be known as the "Man of the Holy Shadow." By his mere presence, all were blessed.

I was once asked by a reporter to describe Sri Gurudev's legacy. Without any hesitation I replied, "His greatest legacy is that he transformed lives and saved souls." With a look, a touch, a word— by his presence alone—bodies were healed, hearts opened, minds expanded. When you looked into his eyes, there was nobody home. It was like gazing through a portal into the center of the universe. And when he looked into yours, you felt he could see everything—that he knew everything you did and didn't do, and everything you would do and wouldn't do. And he loved you anyway. That, in itself, was the greatest source of healing: the power of love.

Many years ago, I went through a difficult period with my health. After a long struggle, I became exhausted—physically, mentally, emotionally, and spiritually. All my efforts to restore my health were to no avail. I cried out to God: "Have you forgotten me? Don't you care about me anymore?" And in utter despair I added, "I'm no longer going to pray to you. I'm not going to talk to you anymore." My main spiritual practice at the time was prayer and inwardly conversing with God. I spoke, trusting that God was listening. The habit was so strong, that the next moment, I looked up and said, "So, what do you think about that?" Then, I had an idea. It was a weekday afternoon. I was in a room with a television. So I said, "I'm going to turn on the TV. If there is anything you wish to tell me, please do so through the television."

I knew that the only thing on at that time were soap operas, so I figured an actor would say something, and I would draw some indirect meaning, and that would be the end of it. Little did I suspect that divine mischief was at play. I turned on the TV, and there was a soap opera—for about ninety seconds. Then the screen went blank, and a banner appeared that read, "A One-Minute Message from God." Suddenly I felt like a thousand eyes were watching me.

I sat bolt upright. When the scene opened, there was a minister seated behind a desk. He began: "I'm going to tell you a story. Once a young mother visited a parish. The priest asked her, 'Mother, you have many children. Which one do you love the most?' The woman reflected a moment and then replied, 'Whoever is away from home, I love them the most until they return. Whoever is ill, I love them the most until they are well.'"

Then, the minister stood up and walked around to the front of the desk. The camera angle changed, so that he now seemed to be gazing directly into my eyes. "So," he said, "if you are having trouble with your health, don't feel that God has forgotten you. He is closer to you now than ever before. And don't stop praying. God wants you to pray to Him. Reach out to God in prayer." The screen went blank. A banner appeared signaling the end of "A One-Minute Message from God," and normal broadcasting resumed.

In that brief interlude, God's love was made visible. It was intimate, reassuring. Whether it was an instance of bizarre synchronicity or divine mystery, I may never know. But the result was that hope was restored, efforts were renewed, and healing ensued. That love is with us always. It fills us, surrounds us, and flows between us. In that ocean of love, the possibilities for healing abound.

Choosing Your Point of View

In the *Talmud*, a sacred text of the Jewish faith, it is written that, "We do not see things as they are; we see things as we are." In other words, in any situation, there are always other points of view.

Swami Satchidananda recounted the following tale told by Sri Ramakrishna, a renowned saint of India: One morning, several people were taking a walk when they came upon a man lying by the side of the road. The first one who saw him said, "That fellow must have spent the whole night in the gambling den, lost all his money, and couldn't reach home, so he fell asleep here." The next person who passed by said, "Poor man, he must be sick. I should probably go for help." The third person decided that the man must have drunk too much and collapsed in a stupor. Then, a fourth person came by and mused, "To a saint, nothing matters. Even if he is lying on the road, he'll just go into *samadhi*. Probably he has transcended physical consciousness." He bowed with reverence and then continued on his walk.

All four saw the same person, but each saw him differently, because each projected something of himself. The world is nothing but our projection. Based on our mental condition, we see things in a certain way and respond accordingly. If we accept this principle, we have a practical approach for maintaining our peace and emotional balance in daily life. No matter what happens, we can always remind ourselves that there are other points of view, and we can try to shift our angle of vision.

Imagine a wheel with spokes emerging from a central hub. They all emanate from the same source and have an integrated function to perform. But if you asked any spoke out at the rim, how to go to the center, each would have a different story to tell. The spoke on top, for example, would say, "You have to go directly south." The one on bottom would say, "Go north." And as time passed and the wheel turned, the perspective at any given point along the rim would change.

Likewise, with the passage of time and the accrual of new experiences, our own views change about different situations. Something we may have opposed at one time becomes the focus of our support at a later date. Our perceptions and reactions are colored by all our past conditioning. We may think we are weighing things neutrally, but in fact, our "scales" are not set to zero. We have been conditioned, our set point has been determined by all our past experiences, including family, friends, environment, education, culture, media, and religious affiliation. It's as if each one of us were fitted with our own particular pair of glasses. We all look out on the same scene, but perceive it very differently and then react accordingly. This sets the stage for turmoil between individuals, as well as social, political and religious conflict in the world.

For the most part, we are not cognizant of all this conditioning as we formulate opinions, pronounce judgments, and decide on courses of action. We don't see the glasses we are wearing, even though everything we do see is filtered through them. Here is where meditation, introspection, and self-analysis can be so helpful. Through regular practice, we begin to understand the type of glasses we are wearing. We learn how to observe the mind and see more clearly how it functions. Habitual patterns are brought into conscious awareness. We can see the once hidden forces and motives that have been driving our attitudes and behaviors. This affords us some distance from what had been automatic modes of functioning, and we are able to see things more neutrally. With this deeper insight comes the capacity to make adjustments.

A little reflection will reveal that what we care most about in any situation are not the bare facts themselves but, rather, how they make us feel. In other words, it's not the external situation that is of primary concern, but our relationship to it. Sometimes we may get discouraged about things we cannot change, all the while ignoring the one thing we, and we alone, can change: our attitude.

Once, the Sufi master Nasrudin decided to plant a flower garden. He worked very diligently and, in due season, a beautiful array of flowers bloomed. But much to his dismay, interspersed among the flowers were many dandelions. Not knowing how to eliminate them, Nasrudin sought the advice of the other gardeners in the village. He tried every remedy they offered, with no success. As a last resort, he traveled to the palace to consult with the royal gardener.

After listening carefully as Nasrudin told of his plight, the gardener offered numerous suggestions, all of which Nasrudin had already tried. Having exhausted all possible solutions, the gardener became very quiet and reflective. When he finally spoke, his advice was simple: "Nasrudin, my friend, learn to love dandelions!"

Everyone's life has its ups and downs. If we allow ourselves to simply go on automatic, it can be challenging at times to maintain a positive perspective. This is where we need to step back, reflect, and analyze. Then we can make good, conscious choices as to how to proceed.

There are a series of statements, known as the "Paradoxical Commandments," that provide a guide for making this sort of attitudinal shift. They were originally written by a man named Kent Keith, when he was a student at Harvard in the 1960s, as part of a booklet for high school student leaders. They enjoin us to always choose what is right and good and true in any circumstance, irrespective of the actions of others. Over the years, variations have been offered, including the one below. At one point, authorship was even attributed to Mother Teresa, because of a version posted on the wall of her children's home in Calcutta.

1. People are often unreasonable, illogical, and self-centered. Forgive them anyway.

2. If you are kind, people may accuse you of selfish, ulterior motives. Be kind anyway.

3. If you are successful, you will win some false friends and some true enemies. Be successful anyway.

4. If you are honest and frank, people may cheat you. Be honest and frank anyway.

5. What you spend years building, someone could destroy overnight. Build anyway.

6. If you find serenity and happiness, people may be jealous. Be happy anyway.

7. The good you do today, people will often forget tomorrow. Do good anyway.

8. Give the world the best you have, and it may never be enough. Give the world the best you have anyway.

9. You see, in the final analysis, it is between you and God. It was never between you and them anyway.

There are times when every one of us may find ourselves dealing with people who seem "unreasonable, illogical, and self-centered." How different might our reactions be if we could shift to the perspective offered in Commandment #9—if we saw everyone and everything as instruments of the Divine, providing the lessons and experiences we need at that very moment.

In France, in the 18th century, there lived a Jesuit Father by the name of Jean Pierre de Caussade. In his insightful classic on spiritual life called *Self-Abandonment to Divine Providence,* he asserted that God is always communicating to us through all the events of our lives, big and small. In the present moment, God's will for us is made clear. As de Caussade stated, "There is no moment at which God does not present himself under the guise of some suffering, some consolation, or some duty. All that occurs within us, around us, and by our means covers and hides his divine action. . . .Could we pierce the veil and were we vigilant and attentive, God would reveal himself continuously to us, and we should rejoice in his action in everything that happens to us."

Instead of accepting our experiences in this way, however, we often pursue our own imaginary concepts of what we think our lives should be like. The result is: Instead of learning the lessons and keeping our peace, we may find ourselves feeling frustrated, victimized, or betrayed.

Swami Satchidananda put it this way: "It's all Your Name. It's all Your Form. It's all Your Deed. And it's all for good." This is, in effect, the ultimate point of view. If we can remember this always, we will have found a most powerful way to change our angle of vision and maintain our peace always.

Finding Your Way to Forgiveness

Forgiveness is a "win-win" approach to life. I once read a story told by Jack Kornfield, a Buddhist meditation teacher. It was about a teenage boy who killed another teenager. The mother of the victim attended the trial. After the conviction, she walked over to the boy who had killed her son and said, "I'm going to kill you."

Several months passed and she began to visit him, bringing food and small gifts. Near the end of his incarceration, she learned that he had nowhere to go. So, she invited him to come live with her and helped him find a job. Then, one day she reminded him of the moment in the courtroom when she said she was going to kill him. She explained that she hadn't wanted her son's killer to remain alive, so she decided to change him. That was why she had been so kind to him. And her plan succeeded; he had changed. So now, since her son was gone and the young man who had killed him was no longer the same, she offered to adopt him and become his mother. With a love that is almost impossible to fathom, she became the mother of the boy who had killed her son.

There's a saying, "To err is human; to forgive is divine." Mahatma Gandhi was once asked how he could put up with all the injustice and cruelty in the world. He responded, "I'm such a scoundrel myself, I have compassion for all the other scoundrels." When we consider our own weaknesses and mistakes and how hard it is for us to change, shouldn't we be more compassionate and forgiving to others? Swami Satchidananda used to say that, when we point a finger of accusation at someone, there are three fingers pointing back at us; and there's one, the thumb, standing up—like God—witnessing everything.

Sri Patanjali, in the *Yoga Sutras,* speaks of *tapas,* which means accepting pain as help for purification. All the difficulties and ordeals make us strong. We are like gold being purified. The problems chip away at the dross in our personalities so that the true gold in us, our divine image, can shine forth. A saintly person once described it this way: "There are two types of people in the world: the saints and the saint-makers." In other words, there are those who are sent to inspire us, and those who come to purify us. So, the next time you start getting annoyed at someone for pushing all your buttons, thank them instead for showing you your weaknesses and helping you to grow stronger.

The *Tirukkural* advises: "At all times put up with the excesses of others; to forget them at once is even better." You may wonder, "How is it possible to forget when someone has wronged you?" There's a story about a spiritual teacher, who, as a boy, had a classmate who treated him very cruelly. Years later, the former classmate came to visit the teacher and was received with much kindness. Perplexed, he questioned the teacher, "Don't you remember how badly I treated you when we were boys?" The teacher gently replied, "I distinctly remember forgetting it!"

Forgiveness is an act of choice. It is not about denying, condoning, or excusing hurtful actions. Rather, it is the letting go of resentment or retaliation, even when they may seem warranted, and offering instead mercy and love. By so doing, we release the past and let go of negative thoughts and feelings. We become unstuck and can move on in our lives. Energy that was tied up within us becomes available for positive, creative endeavors. Relationships are healed, and we, too, are healed. Forgiveness and healing are linked.

I once met a woman who, twenty years prior, had been diagnosed with terminal liver cancer. As she was about to undergo aggressive therapy in the hospital, she began to reflect: "Maybe I'm going to die from this, but I don't want to die like this." She left the hospital and rented a small cabin. For sustenance, she took steamed vegetables and broth. And every day, she visualized filling herself with forgiveness and letting go of anger. That was her entire treatment protocol. Little by little, she felt her strength return. Within a year, she returned home and resumed her work. Today, decades later, she is leading a healthy, dynamic life.

Consider the alternative: We hold on to feelings of anger, resentment, and betrayal and make our lives miserable. These negative feelings poison our systems and set the stage for serious illness. In Chinese medicine, for example, liver problems are associated with anger. If we cling to our pain, to the wrongs we feel we have suffered, we build walls around our hearts. We imprison ourselves and feel the agony of separation, loneliness, and alienation. It's as if we shut our windows and doors and then cry that we can't see the Light.

In speaking of forgiveness, the *Holy Bible* says: "Forgive us our trespasses as we forgive those who trespass against us." When we forgive others, the spirit of forgiveness flows through us, and we, too, receive the benefit. It's like using a funnel to transfer honey from one vessel to another: the funnel also gets the sweetness. We transfer the honey of divine forgiveness to another and we, too, are forgiven.

Forgiveness issues occur on three levels. First, there are the people or circumstances that we need to forgive. Next, there are those from whom we need to seek forgiveness. Lastly, we may need to forgive ourselves for perceived weaknesses or failures. The following exercises offer some suggestions on how to proceed.

Forgiveness Exercise #1

This exercise is designed to inspire you to forgive others. I discovered it on the Internet, and it has been very illuminating when we've done it in workshops. Begin by purchasing a bag of potatoes. Next, make a list of every person or situation you have not forgiven. For each entry on your list, place one potato in a sack. Carry that sack with you wherever you go for one week. Physically, you will feel the burden, and that pales compared to the subtle energy drain on your system caused by all the grievances and unresolved issues you are carrying. After some time, the potatoes may even start to mold and rot. Then, you'll get a glimpse of how this inner fermentation is preventing you from experiencing the divine fragrance within.

Forgiveness Exercise #2

This exercise is designed to enable you to ask forgiveness from those whom you may have harmed in any way. Asking forgiveness, along with sincere repentance, can be a source of healing—both for you as well as your relationships. Swami Satchidananda addressed this point when speaking about reversing cancer. He said, if you want to heal the body, you need to burn out the karma that caused the problem. To burn out the karma, do a lot of repentance. If you know whom you hurt, go to that person and ask forgiveness. If you don't know what you did or, if it's not possible to contact them anymore, mentally ask for forgiveness. You could even place a picture of the individual before you and offer your prayers in that way. By such actions, you can purge negative karma and reduce suffering in your life.

Forgiveness Exercise #3

This exercise is designed to foster compassion toward ourselves. Sometimes, it's easier to forgive others than ourselves. We can be our own toughest critic and judge. Many years back, when I was living at Yogaville West in Lake County, California, I was troubled by an interaction that had occurred with a guest several years before. There's a saying in the Hindu tradition: *"Atithi Devo Bhava,"* which means, "Treat the guest as God." The Divine comes to the home in the form of a guest. On one occasion, I had not been very gracious to a visitor, and every time I sat to meditate, remembrance of that event flashed through my mind and disrupted the sitting.

One day, burdened and frustrated in this way, I came up with a plan. I couldn't go to the person to apologize, as I did not know how to contact them. So, I decided to design a penance for myself to be executed over the course of a month, as an act of atonement. It was the coldest winter in recorded history, and I had a demanding job at the local newspaper. I decided to fast one full day every week. It was challenging, but doable. In my heart, I asked God to please accept my penance.

Those were the pioneer days of the IYI. We had little in the way of financial resources and lived very frugally; rarely did we have special treats. The room I occupied was in a solitary location, not frequented by others. With some difficulty, I completed the month. On the very last day, when I returned to my room, there was a surprise awaiting me. In the center of my altar, wrapped in gold, was a huge piece of chocolate! I took it as a sign that my penance had been accepted.

We all make mistakes as we wend our way on life's journey. We needn't get stuck in the past, or mired in resentment or despair. Instead, we can learn the lessons, make amends, resolve never to make the same mistakes again, and then do our best to move forward with greater insight, compassion, and humility. We are the ones that forge the chains that bind us, and we also hold the keys to set ourselves free. Forgiveness is one of those master keys. If we use it, the love and light in our lives will grow ever brighter.

TRANSMISSION

Passing the Torch

The ancient Indian scriptures refer to four types of charity or ways we can help one another in life: *anna dhanam, svarna dhanam, vidya dhanam,* and *jnana dhanam.* The first is an offering of food (*anna*), but that only gives satisfaction for a short while, and then more food is needed. The second is the gift of money (*svarna*), but that, too, is limited in what it can provide. The third way is to equip people with knowledge (*vidya*) through education. Then, they can take care of their needs themselves and are not dependent on the charity of others. But the greatest gift we can give is that of spiritual wisdom (*jnana*). Once established in that, peace, happiness, and divine prosperity are assured. That is the gift that Yoga has to offer.

The sacred teachings of Yoga have been passed from guru to disciple, from teacher to student, for millennia. They are a time-tested and proven means to spiritual awakening. As a student or teacher of Yoga, you are a link in this chain of transmission. For most people, the point of entry on this journey is usually Hatha Yoga, finding relief from the pains and stresses of everyday life. After getting a taste of the benefits, many are drawn to the deeper teachings, seeking the permanent release from all suffering that comes when spiritual wisdom dawns.

To become good teachers, we must first be good students. Swami Satchidananda spoke of three "Ds," qualities that would enable us to be good students and ensure success in all our undertakings: discipline, devotion, and dedication.

Discipline entails being regular and consistent in our practice. If we want to go deep, we need to remain focused and not get distracted. Devotion comes when we believe in what we are doing, when our doubts get dispelled and our questions are answered. Then, we can pursue our practice enthusiastically, with unwavering conviction.

The final "D" is dedication. As a student, we study, practice, and experience the benefits. At a certain point, we are ready to share the journey and to dedicate time and energy in the service of others. We may choose to become teachers but, even if we don't, our very presence begins to convey the spirit and message of Yoga. We walk in peace and serve with love wherever life takes us. In that way, we carry the torch of Yoga that has been passed from time immemorial into the world around us—providing comfort, restoring hope, and lifting spirits—making the world a better place with every breath, every thought, every step we take.

The Transmission Equation

For thirty-two years, I had the great good fortune to sit at the feet of my spiritual Guru, Sri Swami Satchidananda. I worshipped and adored there, struggled and resisted, celebrated and mourned. There were happy times and sad times, countless comings and goings, many ups and downs—and through it all, he remained the same: peaceful, balanced, patient, and loving—always ready to forgive and forget, ever there to comfort and guide.

When he first arrived in America, Swami Satchidananda was surrounded by a group of unkempt, undisciplined souls. He was warned against associating with those "hippies," those "pigs," and told that all respectable people would leave if he continued to do so. But he had the vision to see the hidden yearnings of their hearts, the tiny flickers of light that were desperately sputtering in the darkness. After a moment's reflection, he replied, "Well, if they are pigs, then I must be a mama pig, because they are my kids." And with infinite tenderness, he began to train them. He not only imparted the highest teachings, but he awakened, quickened, the Spirit within us. We not only learned about spiritual life, the miracle was that we practiced it.

There aren't words big enough, deep enough, strong enough, or sweet enough to describe the relationship with the guru. With a word, a touch, or a glance, he could remove an obstacle, dispel the darkness, and restore peace to the most troubled heart. All you had to do was to present your plight before him. He would listen patiently as every last detail was conveyed. Then, after a few moments of silence, you would hear that precious, "Hmm," the sign of divine comprehension and dispensation. With that single, "Hmm," you knew that everything—no matter how complex or convoluted the problem might seem—would be resolved. And it always was.

"Gu" represents darkness; "ru" means remover. The guru is the one who removes the darkness of ignorance. He or she is the grace of God in human form, come to free the soul of all sorrow and suffering. The guru is the one who has realized the higher truth and can guide others to that experience.

There's a type of puzzle that involves a maze, and the object is to figure out how to get from the starting point to the end goal. If you make a wrong turn, you're likely to wind up in a dead end, or you'll find yourself circling the goal again and again, never able to reach it. In a way, each of us lives in a self-created maze, the result of countless eons of accumulated karma. The guru is the one who can guide us at those crucial junctures and crossroads along the way. It's a mysterious journey, where the seeker is tested and tempted, refined and purified. We're trying to enter a realm that is beyond the mind and senses, to pierce through the veil of illusory names and forms, and experience the underlying, never-changing reality. There are no maps and few signposts, and things aren't always what they seem.

In the *Holy Bible*, we read that the devil, himself, can appear disguised as an angel of light. We may seem to be making progress, while all that is growing is our arrogance and sense of self-importance. At other times, everything may seem to be falling apart, but our humility, faith, and surrender to God may be deepening. It's difficult to evaluate spiritual matters with material eyes, and so the guidance of a spiritual master is of inestimable value to help keep us on the right track.

The master, however, is only one part of the equation. Equally important is the disciple. The *Bhagavad Gita* describes the qualities of a good student. Verse 4.34 states: "If you seek enlightenment from those who have realized the truth, prostrate before them, question them, and serve them. Only then are you open to receive their teachings of sacred knowledge." Prostrate means to be humble. Knowledge flows from the teacher to the student when there is humility. It's like water flowing from one vessel to another. If you place one beneath the other and connect them with a hose, the water will flow to the lower one.

Through questioning, you show your open-mindedness and eagerness to learn. You get your doubts and confusion cleared. Through service, the teachings are put into practice. You become aware of your weaknesses and learn how to correct them. You show your sincerity, commitment, and gratitude for all that you have received. You may hear many nice lectures about *ahimsa* (non-violence) and agree with it in principle—but if you then go and slam a door, or unthinkingly swat a fly, or speak harshly to a friend, you see how far you still have to go to integrate non-violence into your life.

The Tamil scriptures speak of three levels of students. The first level is like a swan or a cow. If you give a swan a bowl of milk mixed with water, it has the capacity to extract the milk, leaving the water behind. Likewise, the topmost student will always glean what is good and valuable in a situation and leave anything undesirable behind. A cow accomplishes the same end, but with a different technique. Initially, it ingests everything while grazing, but then it brings it up again, chews it well, and spits out anything undesirable. What remains is the good and nutritious food to become a part of its system.

The second level of student is compared to a parrot or the earth. If you teach a parrot to say "Ram, Ram," it will say "Ram, Ram." Teach it to say, "Poppycock," and it will say, "Poppycock." In either case, it will have no idea of the meaning behind the utterance. In like manner, if you plant an apple seed in the earth, you will get an apple tree; a mango seed will yield a mango tree. This type of student can only recount what he heard and never really understands the teachings.

The third level of student is likened either to a goat, a buffalo, a pot with holes, or a tea strainer. A goat can be restless. It will sample all sorts of things; eat a little here, then a little there. In this, it resembles students who don't stick to one spiritual path; they are easily attracted and distracted by different teachings and don't go deep in their practice. If a buffalo comes to a clear pool of water, it will first roll around in the water, stirring up all the mud, and only then will it drink. Likewise, for some students, no sooner do they hear the teachings, than they get muddled in their minds. A pot with holes represents the proverbial "in one ear, out the other" approach to learning: nothing of value is retained. At least that is better than the last category, the tea strainer. This type of student is the opposite of the topmost level of student. He only retains the dregs; if anything undesirable comes along, that is what engages his interest. We can all look at ourselves and determine in what category we belong and how we can improve.

For students of a spiritual master, a time comes when the guru is no longer in the physical body. The question then becomes: How to continue to feel his or her presence and guidance in one's life? Consider the following: During all the years that Sri Gurudev traveled the globe, in the midst of all the comings and goings, something always remained. It was invisible, yet somehow tangible. His Spirit abided with us always. And that is no less true today than it was then.

Rather than say Sri Gurudev is no longer in the physical body, I think it is more correct to say that he is no longer in his *limited* body. His consciousness is everywhere, and he can function unfettered by physical limitations. Several months ago, I had just completed a big project at the *ashram*. Before retiring for the night, I was reflecting that no one realized all the planning, effort, and work that had been involved. Suddenly I felt a presence, which seemed to approach and then surround me. I clearly heard Sri Gurudev's voice. "Hmm," he said, "so *you're* the one doing all this." It was a perfect and playful reminder of the true spirit of Karma Yoga (the path of selfless service), and how each and every one of us is but an instrument in the hands of the Divine.

The Buddhists speak of the Triple Treasure: the Buddha (or spiritual master), the *Dharma* (the teaching), and the *Sangha* (the community of seekers who follow the teaching). The teacher comes to light the way and is an embodiment of the teachings. We cannot be in his or her physical presence always, but the teachings are eternal. Through our observance of the teachings and dedicated practice, we stay attuned to the teacher.

Sometimes, however, our lives may get so busy or our minds so cluttered, that we may forget the teachings. Then, the *sangha* is there to help us remember. The *sangha* is an expression of the expanded body of the teacher. By ourselves, we may not be able to stay the course and surmount all the obstacles that may arise, but, together, we can make it to the spiritual goal. We can draw inspiration, strength, and guidance from one another. Just like in a family, the more mature or experienced members can help the younger ones along.

Sri Gurudev walked in our midst for so many years, and now he continues to dance in our hearts. The relationship with the guru is eternal. The power of the guru's presence and the wisdom of the guru's teachings are imprinted on the soul forever. His or her Spirit remains accessible to one and all. Sri Gurudev, himself, gave this assurance when he said, "Remember, you will never be without me; never, never, never! The body may go, but I am always with you. Always!"

What We Seek Is Who We Are

At a meeting with his California students, Swami Satchidananda once playfully remarked: "On the East Coast I'm mining diamonds, and on the West Coast I'm mining gold." "How beautiful," I thought, "Together we will form a crown—a living tribute to the treasured teachings of Yoga." But the deeper significance of his words became clearer over time.

Sri Gurudev's main residence was on the East Coast. Coal is mined in that part of the country, and diamonds are formed when coal is subjected to constant pressure over a long time. Sri Gurudev's constant presence, watchful eye and hands-on involvement in the life of his disciples constituted the pressure needed to effect brilliant transformation.

He came to California for visits. Eventually, we purchased a winter residence for him near the Santa Barbara *ashram*. So, his stays were longer; but, still, we did not see him on a daily basis. When we did see him, though, there was a special closeness, caring, and connection; you knew he was your very own. The time may have been shorter by chronological measure, but the intensity and activity were so concentrated, that months were packed into minutes, years were packed into days. We were like gold being purified—dipped into the crucible of his love and heated to the boiling point. As we cooled, layer after layer of impurities were eliminated.

The spiritual atmosphere in those early days was amazing. Our eyes were opened, spirits ignited, hope restored. A new way of life was shown to us, and we were eager to bring it into manifestation. In 1969, four of Sri Gurudev's close students packed up their belongings and headed west to open centers in San Francisco and Los Angeles. A beautiful Victorian mansion was found in San Francisco, perfectly structured and situated for an Integral Yoga Institute. There was one problem, however. We had little money for a down payment and needed generous terms for the mortgage. And at the same time, there was a wealthy young couple offering to buy the house for cash. The owner was a retired Army officer, so you can imagine what she must have thought looking at us, with our long tresses, bell-bottoms and bangles. There is a verse from the *Tirukkural* that states: "What is not destined to be yours will not stay even if you guard it; what is destined to be yours will not leave even if you cast it aside." Some sort of destiny must have been in play, because she decided to sell the house to us, and 770 Dolores Street became the home for the Integral Yoga Institute of San Francisco.

The early beginnings of the New Age Movement that swept the country—and later the world—can be traced to the San Francisco Bay Area. The San Francisco IYI was well positioned to serve as a fertile womb for this rebirth of spirituality. Its outreach programs extended throughout the city and to neighboring counties. Classes were taught at schools, colleges, and hospitals; at the *San Francisco Chronicle* newspaper, the YWCA, the Sierra Club, and the jail; for the Department of Social Services and the Lighthouse for the Blind and at many other venues. Additionally, the IYI joined with members of other spiritual groups in the area—including 3HO and the Sufi Order—to found "Meeting of the Ways." We had monthly meetings, our own radio show, and held a big annual event, providing a forum for the teachers of our respective groups. It was a wonderful opportunity to network, to get to know one another better, and to share from the richness of our varied traditions.

The high point each year for the California devotees was our annual retreat. In 1970 and 1971, it was held at a camp in the Santa Cruz Mountains. Hundreds attended. Every morning and evening, Sri Gurudev would expound on the teachings of Raja Yoga. In that brisk, rustic setting, our lives found new meaning and direction.

Then, one year we received news that Sri Gurudev would not be able to attend. We were shaken, despondent. We depended on the retreat to re-charge our batteries. We thought that Gurudev had something special that we lacked, and when we were with him, he gave some of it to us. So, it was with some disappointment that we decided to conduct the retreat anyway. We observed silence and maintained the same schedule. We came together for meditation, conducted Hatha Yoga classes, and senior disciples gave discourses on the teachings. And much to our surprise, we got it, even though Sri Gurudev was not physically present. It was a dramatic demonstration of the key teaching of Yoga—that what we are seeking is who we are in truth. To experience that, we need to calm the mind and go within—not look for someone else to give it to us. We learned firsthand the power of the teachings and the purpose of *sangha.*

Recognizing the value of *sangha* and living together in community, we established our first *ashram* in 1972 in Lake County, California. It was called "Yogaville West" and was situated at a former hot springs resort, known as Seigler Springs. The place was equipped for summer habitation only, and we were about to face the coldest winter in recorded history. But we were equal to the challenge! Someone got the idea of securing old oil drums and converting them into wood-burning stoves. We dutifully followed all the instructions, but after considerable effort, all we got was a lot of smoke and very little heat. On any given day, you could find half a dozen *ashramites* huddled in the cooler to get warm. Yes, you read it correctly: the cooler. I have fond memories of seeing the kitchen mother using a hammer and pick to pry loose some honey from its tin.

Sri Gurudev, however, had other ways to heat us up. He decided that this was the year we were to learn how to control the tongue, because he said, "If you can control the tongue, you can attain total self-mastery." According to the Yoga teachings, we have five organs of sense and five organs of action. The sense organs are: the eyes, ears, nose, touch receptors in the skin, and tongue as the organ of taste. The organs of action are: the hands, feet, organ of elimination, organ of procreation, and tongue as the organ of speech. The tongue is unique in that it is the only organ that is both an organ of action and an organ of sense: it talks and tastes. It thus plays a pivotal role in our subtle physiology. So, we were to observe silence and have simple meals consisting of two or three items.

In this manner, we entered the fire of *tapasya*, engaging in self-discipline, while accepting some discomfort as an aid toward purification. Many good lessons and spiritual growth resulted. We were pioneers, adventurers in the realm of Spirit, and no task was too difficult, no challenge too great, that we didn't embrace it with fervor.

The first pre-*sannyas* (pre-monastic) initiation was held there during a retreat in 1973. I can still recall the moment that the first group of pre-*sannyasis* emerged, heads shaven, necks adorned with orange scarves to indicate their commitment to a life of total renunciation. They were absolutely radiant. I kept gazing from Sri Gurudev to them, and then back again to Sri Gurudev. The scarves looked like they came from his orange robe; the new initiates looked like they were emanations of his Spirit. Suddenly, whatever was holding me back from pursuing the monastic path was released. It felt like something within me snapped free, and I knew that I, too, would soon embrace that path.

Costly maintenance problems necessitated our selling that property, but we had the good fortune to later purchase sixty-five acres in Santa Barbara. This former avocado and lemon orchard was to become our new *ashram*. There were only two buildings on the property: a hundred-year-old farmhouse that had once been a Pony Express stop and a barn. The house served as the women's quarters, kitchen, dining hall, and offices; and the barn housed the men and became our *satsang* hall. We ran a falafel stand in the neighboring university town of Isla Vista and operated a food distribution business, known as Prana Produce. We also purchased a beautiful home for Sri Gurudev, which he named "*La Paz*," in the neighboring town of Montecito. For several years, he wintered there, affording us many opportunities to work with him directly, attend his *satsangs*, and delight in numerous celebrations and outings.

One of my most cherished memories in Santa Barbara was the visit of Sivaya Subramuniyaswami, a dear friend of Sri Gurudev and well-known Hindu spiritual leader, with some of his disciples. We all crowded into the house together for a meeting of the two great masters. At one point, Sivaya Subramuniyaswami looked around the room and tenderly gazed at each one of us. Then, he turned to Sri Gurudev and said, "Swamiji, I can tell that they are your disciples. They all have your eyes."

144

Sri Gurudev first considered building the Light Of Truth Universal Shrine (LOTUS) at the Santa Barbara *ashram*. Plans were drawn, and meetings were held with the Planning Commission. However, some of the neighbors were concerned about having such a unique-looking shrine in their neighborhood. Sri Gurudev said that LOTUS was to be our special gift to the world, and that he didn't want to build it where even one person objected. So, the project was shifted to the East coast. We sold the *ashram* property, consolidated our resources, and moved to Virginia to help build the *ashram* there.

Satchidananda Ashram–Yogaville in Virginia has grown from those simple beginnings to become a thriving Yoga community—home to hundreds of aspirants and host to many thousands of guests and students every year. For many years, it served as the main residence for Sri Gurudev. Then, in August 2002, Sri Gurudev entered *Mahasamadhi*, the termed used to describe the final conscious exit from the body by an enlightened soul.

In the atmosphere of loss and grief that surrounded the passing of Sri Gurudev, memories of the early days in California with him filled my mind. I recalled that retreat many years ago when he was physically absent, but the teachings were transmitted beautifully and, together, we created a space in which the peace and power of Yoga were experienced. In that moment, my heart knew that the transmission of these sacred teachings would continue—and that more and more, we would come to realize that what we seek is who we are.

Going Fast, Getting Nowhere

There is a story about an avid seeker who pursued his practice with such intensity that he even neglected to eat or sleep. His teacher became concerned and gently cautioned him to slow down, but the student persisted. Finally, the teacher decided to intervene more emphatically and inquired, "Why are you always in such a hurry? Why are you driving yourself so hard?"

The student replied, "I am determined to reach enlightenment. I don't want to waste a minute."

"Aha," said the teacher, "you seem to be under the impression that enlightenment is somehow in front of you, and if you rush, you'll catch up to it. Did you ever consider the possibility that it might be behind you, and if you just stayed still, you would experience it? Maybe, you are running away from it!"

Years ago, I attended a major Yoga conference. It was held at a beautiful hotel; over a thousand people participated. The conference was wonderful in so many ways. It was obvious that an enormous amount of time, effort, and expertise went into planning every detail. People came from all over the country to share their knowledge, practice, and experience. It was a time to connect, explore, and rejoice together. For several days, everyone immersed themselves in Yoga.

There were many sessions throughout the day, numerous offerings in each time slot. As a workshop drew to a close, the presenters and students alike would quickly gather their mats and cushions, and then dash to the next event. Between sessions, the Yoga bazaar was the place to go, filled with books, tapes, props, clothing, jewelry, and all sorts of Yoga-related accessories.

As the days unfolded, the conference began to reflect more and more the hectic, outer-oriented pace of modern life. There was little time or space provided for the participants to enjoy the peace that is the goal of the practices. Little things could have made a big difference—like a dedicated room that was always available for meditation. Or imagine what it would have been like if, once or twice a day, there were five minutes of silence when everyone—wherever they were—paused and meditated. What a tremendous vibration of peace could have been generated—for the benefit of all those at the conference and for the rest of the world as well!

In the West, we know how to achieve. We pride ourselves on our ability to multi-task. We "do lunch" with business associates, frequent fast-food vendors, and quaff energy drinks on the run. We even organize and schedule our children's playtime. We know that stress is a major factor in disease, yet our lives are laced with it. We know how to achieve; our challenge is to learn how to relax. Yoga is ideally suited to enable us to meet that challenge with resounding success—that is, if in the name of Yoga, we don't create similar conditions to the ones we are trying to overcome.

The science of Yoga can be traced to ancient roots and simpler times, to a traditional culture in India. In the last century, this science was transplanted to the West. Whenever you have a cultural transplant, it is inevitable that after some time, the values and methods of the host begin to impact and influence the new arrival. That is what we are seeing today. On the positive side, there is a genuine integration of Yoga in the West. We are making it our own, adapting it in creative ways to meet the needs of our society. Yoga studios can be found everywhere; classes are taught in schools, businesses, churches, hospitals, gyms, prisons, and all sorts of venues. As Yoga is becomingly increasingly popular, available, and relevant to modern needs, it might be useful for us to look at how the high-pressure, materialistic, competitive ethos of our society may be seeping into our approach to Yoga as well.

In our diverse and fluid culture, with instant communication powered by the internet, a global repository of information is available at a keystroke. We can watch a Yoga class on YouTube or attend a webinar offering spiritual instruction. We have come to value the quick and convenient, and sometimes pass over that which requires more time and effort. Information sometimes gets mistaken for knowledge, and knowledge masquerades as wisdom. With respect to spiritual growth, Swami Satchidananda used to say, "The slower path is the safer one. Slow and steady wins the race." It can be hard to keep that sentiment in the forefront, when the other aspects of our lives seem to be rushing ahead at such great speed.

Traditionally, Yoga was learned in the context of the guru-disciple relationship. The disciple often lived with and served the guru for many years. The guru, in turn, instructed and transmitted the teachings to the worthy student. The teachings came with the authority of the guru, backed by the established lineage that he or she represented.

Today, with so much information readily available, Yoga practitioners sometimes opt instead for a more eclectic approach, rather than aligning themselves with one lineage. In the beginning, when we're searching for the teachings that are right for us, it can be very helpful to check out various schools, to explore and experiment. But once we have found what works for us, it's good to settle in and go deep. When we begin to pick and choose from various schools, we may not arrive at an integrated or well-rounded practice. We may gravitate toward that which feels good, rather than what is truly good for us, thus reinforcing our strengths and never fully addressing our weaknesses. We might adroitly avoid that which we most need. Cross-currents from different approaches might dilute the benefits we could receive.

It is my belief that all the great masters included checks and balances in their systems. Some of these built-in protective measures may have been directly articulated; others may have been subtly threaded throughout the whole body of teaching. They could take the form of lifestyle guidelines, sequences, contraindications, or directions as to when to practice or how to develop the practice. When we pick and choose, we may unknowingly overlook some of these crucial pointers.

The aim of spiritual practice is to make the mind steady. When the mind is calm and clear, it resembles a pristine lake. We can see through the waters to the depths of our being and experience our true nature, perfect peace and joy. If in the very name of practice, we keep changing what we are doing, we subtly encourage the restless tendency of the mind. So, our method becomes counter-productive to our goal.

This may bring up a number of questions: If we're interested in spiritual growth, then what can change and what should remain the same? How do we keep our practice alive and engaging without going off course? How do we stay true to our tradition and, at the same time, remain relevant to the times in which we live? As teachers, how can we equip ourselves to best serve the special populations that we teach?

Here are some reflections that are humbly offered for consideration. If we wish to look to various schools to augment our practice, it might be useful to first ask ourselves why we are doing this. If the answer is boredom or the allure of something new, different, or popular, these are usually tricks of the mind and distractions. If the answer is we don't feel we are receiving proper guidance or support, we can try reaching out to other teachers and practitioners within our own tradition. If we feel frustrated at a seeming lack of progress, perhaps what is needed is more patience and perseverance on our part. If we try some other practice, we may come up against the same sort of situation down the road. Swami Satchidananda compared the spiritual path to digging a well. If we want to reach water, we need to stay in one place and keep digging. If we keep switching, we may dig thousands of feet and never succeed. If we want to attain the goal of Yoga, we need to go deep in our practice.

On the other hand, if we are well established in our practice, at some point, we may wish to broaden our understanding in specific ways. As Yoga teachers, we may be serving populations with special needs: like children, seniors, military veterans, or people facing health challenges. Different schools may have developed specialties in certain areas and have methods that are particularly suited for the people we are called to serve. I think the important thing to consider is whether or not those teachings are in keeping with the spirit and approach of our tradition. Both in our own practice and when serving others, we want there to be a clear and consistent experience.

Ancient wisdom and modern technology have come together today to provide us with extraordinary opportunities for spiritual inquiry and growth. We can connect with fellow seekers and teachers all over the globe for inspiration, instruction, and support. The world is truly our village now. We can also gather to immerse ourselves in Yoga programs, retreats, and celebrations. In such settings, a moment shared—through a look, a touch, a word—can be the impetus for profound spiritual insight and discovery. We can make the most of all that is available. Instead of going fast and getting nowhere, together, we can find our way to true peace and happiness, and rest in the "now-here."

Mainstream Yoga

It was in 1966 that Swami Satchidananda came to the West. Yoga was seen as quite exotic back then. Many were experimenting with it as a natural high. Some were trying it out as a new fad, following the lead of the Beatles and other pop culture icons. Others were just drifting, disillusioned by the greed and corruption they saw in society and the politics that had produced the Vietnam War, and they embraced Yoga as an alternative lifestyle.

At a time when many were exploring altered realities, there he stood rooted in the ultimate reality. It was a time when many great masters were being drawn here, attracted by the awakening aspiration of the youth. Their spiritual light ignited the flickering flame within the hearts of those young seekers, many of whom spent the ensuing years immersing themselves in the study and practice of Yoga. That's when Yoga began to flourish in the West. It was the first big wave.

There's a story about the Chinese sage, Chuang-Tzu, who once had a dream in which he was a butterfly. When he woke up, he didn't know for sure if before he had been a man dreaming he was a butterfly, or if now, he was a butterfly dreaming he was a man. Likewise, we're all caught in a dream of our own creation. The influx of these great masters set us on a journey of awakening.

Now, imagine for a moment what would happen if you were in the middle of a dream, and suddenly an enlightened being, someone who is fully awake, entered it. I once had a dream in which I was giving a lecture to a roomful of people. As I was talking, Sri Gurudev entered and sat down directly in front of me. The quality of his presence was different from everything else in the dream; it felt as if he had really dropped in to check on me. As he sat there watching me, with perfect, unwavering attention, I became totally unnerved. I forgot what I was saying. All my mental constructs began to evaporate. That gaze of pure awareness, of perfect knowing, produced profound changes in me. He didn't have to *do* anything. He just was there, in the dream, watching.

As I stood there stuttering and stammering, one by one, everyone in the audience began to leave, and I thought, "I better do something quick." And then the thought came, "Why not talk about Raja Yoga? I've done that so often, I could do it in my sleep." So I proceeded to give an introductory talk on Raja Yoga, which had the effect of pulling me out of the dream into the waking state. When I awoke, I was still giving the talk.

In a similar manner, Sri Gurudev entered into the life we were dreaming. Among all that we saw and experienced in the world, we could sense a definite difference in the quality of his presence. It may have been indefinable, but it was nonetheless undeniable and irresistible. He entered into our dream like the dawning of a great sun, and we began to stir from our slumber.

During that period, several hundred people would typically attend our Integral Yoga retreats. In California, those early retreats were held at Camp Kennolyn in the Santa Cruz Mountains. We came from many places for diverse reasons, but together, we plunged into five days of intensive practice. No matter what our intention in coming, we left filled with the prospect of new possibilities—another way of seeing, thinking, acting, living, being.

I remember one such retreat well. One afternoon, around 3:00 p.m., we had a walking meditation. The leader set out with several hundred people in single file behind him. Several hours passed, and the staff gathered in the dining hall for dinner, only to find it totally empty. This was serious; no one missed meals in those days, so we immediately became concerned.

It was dusk; darkness was quickly descending. We began to compare notes about when we had last seen anyone, and then, before our startled gaze, the retreatants began trickling in, still silent and in single file. They had been lost in the Santa Cruz Mountains for three hours. They marched in peacefully, just as if everything had transpired according to plan. It was beautiful to behold, and in a way, conveys the spirit that characterized that first big wave of Yoga in the West.

Today, we are witnessing another big wave: Yoga has gone mainstream. A search for "Yoga" on the Internet will yield over 130 million results. Articles about it appear in leading newspapers and magazines. Classes and studios can be found everywhere. Yoga clothes, props, and accessories have become a booming business.

Along with this growing presence of Yoga in society, we've also been seeing the departure, in physical form, of many of the great teachers who came to lead the way. Since ancient times, the Yoga teachings have been passed from master to disciple in an unbroken chain of succession, and it seems like the torch is being passed to our generation. The important questions before us are: Are we ready to carry it? Will we do our utmost to tend that flame so it will continue to shine brightly for generations yet to come? Will we retain the vision, fervor, and dedication that our teachers inspired within us?

This is the challenge before us, and it is also the need of the hour. The entire world is yearning for peace. That abiding peace that everyone is seeking can never be negotiated by politicians, nor guaranteed by treaties. It certainly can't be won on the battlefield. That peace is the purpose, the gift that Yoga has to offer. Yoga provides teachings and techniques that will enable us to experience supreme peace and then share it with others. But that purpose is not always recognized.

In the midst of Yoga's growing popularity, we need to find ways to communicate its higher purpose and keep that in the forefront, so that more superficial interests don't intrude. A well-known Yoga teacher visited Satchidananda Ashram and was talking about a conversation he had with a few students. They were complaining of injuries they had suffered from attending Yoga classes that were too strenuous for them, and yet, said they were still going to the same classes. When he asked them why they would continue doing something that had caused them injury, they replied that they liked the clothes worn in the classes.

In the year before his *Mahasamadhi*, Sri Gurudev said it was time for the Yoga community worldwide to go beyond the physical level and to explore the deeper teachings of Yoga. We are being called now to gently guide our students to that deeper level. In order to do that, we need to experience it ourselves. That means we need to walk our spiritual path with renewed conviction and commitment, patience and perseverance, faith and courage. As we dedicate ourselves to our practice, the path will unfold before us.

Life is fleeting like a dream. Time is short. So, let us commit to doing all that we can to realize that supreme peace and then share it with one and all. In this way, we will carry the torch of Yoga in the spirit with which it was passed and it will continue to light the way for those seeking greater health, happiness, and true fulfillment in life.

The Yoga of Teaching

Beginning in the 1960s, there was a tremendous wave of enlightened masters who came to the West to impart the teachings of Yoga. Their coming was heralded by singular great souls who taught in the early 1900s, like Paramahansa Yogananda and Swami Vivekananda. Most of these teachers came from India. There was a distinct spiritual vibration one felt in their presence. Their ability to elucidate and demonstrate the Yoga teachings and practices was awe-inspiring. Thousands immersed themselves in Yoga.

Students were attracted, and organizations were established. Students were trained, so that the teachings could be disseminated. Today in the West, we don't see the same sort of influx of realized masters. What we do have are Yoga teachers from various traditions who have devoted the past decades to study and practice, and have gone deep on the spiritual path. They bring their knowledge, experience, and insight to the teaching of Yoga, as well as the blessings of the great masters who trained them.

The transmission of spiritual teachings is a privilege and an art. It involves skillfully communicating what we have garnered over the years so that others can reap the benefits as well. There are four key factors that can enhance and ensure the effectiveness of this process: inspiration, information, motivation, and transformation. When they come together, a dynamic environment for exploration, practice, and growth is created in which genuine spiritual unfolding can occur.

Inspiration

People are inspired by not only what you say, but by who you are. They are quick to observe if your presence and manner embody the message you expound. If they experience tranquility and clarity, ease and poise, in the way you speak, act, or move about, it reinforces their confidence in the teachings and gives them hope that they, too, can experience similar benefits. What you have to offer is deemed authentic, valuable, and attainable.

Teach what you love and practice what you teach. This will enliven and give authority to all that you say. Share from your heart, and you will reach the hearts of others. Do so with patience, kindness, and respect for the uniqueness and integrity of each individual's process and path.

When you teach Yoga, something is imparted from the depths of who you are, from your own experience, and that is possible only if you practice sincerely and regularly. The *Yoga Sutras* states that practice must be done for a long time, without break, and in all earnestness in order to become firmly grounded. Such practice becomes a crucible in which spiritual insight crystallizes. We can only give to others that which we ourselves have. So, to be a good teacher, we first need to be good students ourselves. Then, with gratitude for all we have received, we can generously offer the fruits of our practice for the comfort, upliftment, and benefit of others.

Gratitude engenders humility. In speaking at Teacher Training graduations, Swami Satchidananda would often describe how wheat grows. A young plant will be green and stand straight up. But as it ripens, it will turn a golden or orange color and bow low. Wisdom and humility go together. Humility should not be confused with lack of confidence or low self-esteem. It means answering the call to serve when it comes, trusting that all you need will be provided at the right time. Sometimes people undergo comprehensive trainings and then are hesitant to teach. They may feel their knowledge is incomplete or have anxiety about getting up in front of a group. It's important to realize and remember that it is not about you—it's about serving those who are guided to attend your class. Trust that there's a reason—invisible patterns of commonality and forces of attraction—that have brought you all together. There are lessons to be learned, gifts to be shared, support to be given.

You don't have to know everything in order to teach; in fact, that would be impossible. In the Hindu pantheon, Sarasvati, the Goddess of wisdom, is shown holding a book in one hand and a *japa mala* (rosary) in another. The message is: If the Goddess of wisdom is still learning and practicing, who are we to feel that our learning will ever be complete? There's also an Indian saying that reflects this truth: "What we have learned is just a lump of clay; what we have yet to learn is the whole earth itself."

One of the best ways to learn is to teach. When you try to explain something to someone else, you can clearly see the gaps in your own understanding. In my own experience, when I review materials to share with others, greater light comes to bear than when I simply study for my own edification. When I discuss the teachings with a group, the insights from others broaden my own perspective—like seeing light reflected from newly revealed facets of a jewel. After class, I note down all I have learned from the session and that becomes part of my personal study guide. The *Holy Bible* states, "Where two or three are gathered together in my name, I am there." Likewise, when people gather in the name of Yoga, seeking greater health and happiness, peace and spiritual growth, the divine power and grace are there to back their efforts.

Information

When people are inspired, they are more receptive to hear what you have to say. Whether you are offering instruction in Hatha Yoga, Raja Yoga, Karma Yoga, Bhakti Yoga, or Jnana Yoga—whether elucidating a scripture or exploring a practice—communicate in a clear manner material that matches the proficiency level and interests of your group. Just as eating too much food, improperly cooked, and at the wrong time will result in indigestion—consider what can be well assimilated and how best to prepare it. Refrain from overfeeding your students. Like good seasoning, let the beauty of your language bring out the greatness of the teachings.

For lectures or discussions, a dry presentation of information rarely holds peoples' attention or engages their participation. A skillful teacher, like a master chef, has a repertoire of techniques that can help spice up any session. By interspersing information with demonstrations, stories, analogies, scriptural references, or relevant examples from everyday life, a rich and varied texture is created.

Stories, in particular, are very helpful when introducing new, abstract, or possibly controversial points. They immediately slow down the pace and shift the atmosphere from the head to the heart. They are like sugarcoated pills that can help people swallow hard-to-digest ideas, allowing time to ruminate on them further. While it may be easy to oppose a teaching, it's less likely that someone will challenge a story. Later on, by recalling the story, they will remember the teaching. Sri Gurudev once told us, "In the future, continue to tell the stories I told. That way, people will know you are my disciples, and they will remember me through you."

True stories, or anecdotes, can be a fount of hope and inspiration. It's natural to feel that if something worked for someone else, it has the potential to work for you as well. This can foster faith in the teachings and engender stronger motivation to practice.

Motivation

As a teacher, you are a link in an eternal chain, with the original teacher, according to the *Yoga Sutras*, being God. The chain continues with each new student who wholeheartedly embraces the spiritual path. Until their inner motivation is awakened, your interest in their progress can provide the necessary external motivation to keep them going. You can suggest weekly goals for practice or specific ways to incorporate the teachings into daily life. Allowing time in class for sharing about their experiences will promote interest and enthusiasm. Sharing about your own spiritual journey can help make the path feel more real and graspable, especially for beginners. It can make the difficult seem doable; the unattainable, accessible; and whatever obstacles may arise, surmountable.

Transformation

The study and practice of Yoga is not about memorization and imitation; it's about integration and transformation. Ultimately, it's about freedom from all suffering and liberation. The teachings are like a recipe book or a map. Reading a recipe for chocolate cake is hardly the same as enjoying a slice. A map of the Grand Canyon cannot possibly convey the grandeur of actually being there. To have the experience, you need to bake the cake or make the journey.

The role of the teacher in this process is to provide the inspiration, information, and motivation to help students find their path and get established in a regular practice. Sri Gurudev likened the teacher to a signpost, whose purpose is to point the way, so the students can make the journey and reach the goal. We can offer our guidance and support, but the transformation, itself, is a mystical process that happens slowly and quietly within the individual. When the time is right, like a butterfly emerging from a cocoon, the beauty of what has been wrought becomes visible for all to see.

Swami Satchidananda: A Lesson in Teaching

In the mid-1970s, I attended a large Yoga conference in Los Angeles with Gurudev. There were a number of gurus invited, so several presentations were scheduled concurrently. About three hundred people showed up for one of Sri Gurudev's talks. I was curious to see what topic he would select and was stunned when he began to speak about *tapasya*, accepting pain as help for purification. This was southern California, and I felt certain that a topic like "Happiness is Your True Nature" or "Follow Your Bliss" would have been more to the audience's liking. I figured he must know what he is doing, because he was a consummate teacher as well as an enlightened master. But as he proceeded, people began to leave—first one by one, then whole rows at a time. I felt distressed, but he continued unperturbed. By the time he finished, there were only a few rows of listeners remaining. Smiling sweetly, he left the stage.

It was a defining moment for me about what it means to be a teacher. It was clear that teaching was not about being popular. It was not about giving people what they seemed to want, but what they truly needed. It was about serving as an instrument in the hands of a higher wisdom. The talk that day may have been delivered for one person whose need in the moment outweighed everyone else's combined.

Over the years since that experience, I have given many talks and conducted many programs. I have come to realize that the immediate response is not always an indicator of the true impact it might have. Sometimes those who have the most objections become the most devoted students later, and those who seem very enthusiastic soon drift to other interests. A really interesting talk may be entertaining, but have no lasting impact. A simpler presentation might be the impetus that changes someone's life. Who's to know? The *Bhagavad Gita* says, "Do the work that comes to you, but don't look for the results."

As teachers, we are there to serve to the best of our ability. May we be ever grateful for the gift of the teachings, for the training and guidance we have received, and for the privilege of sharing this with others. May all the great teachers who came before us continue to light the way and shower their blessings, so we may walk with integrity, serve with humility, and, ultimately, attain the highest realization.

GLOSSARY

Sanskrit Words, Other Terms, and Names
with References to the *Yoga Sutras of Patanjali*

Note on Sanskrit transliteration: In order to make the Sanskrit more accessible to a wider audience, we have decided not to employ the diacritical marks. We have used a method that should help facilitate a close pronunciation of the words by a western reader. Also, in keeping with the trend to anglicize Sanskrit, we have added "s" to certain words to make them plural.

Abhinivesha — clinging to life; one of the five *kleshas* (See *sutras*: 2.3, 2.9)

Advaita — non-dualism; philosophy that reality is beyond that which appears dualistic and changing, and is actually one and unchanging

Agami — karma being developed in the present; *kriyamana*

Ahamkara — ego feeling, or I-ness feeling

Ahimsa — non-violence; one of the *yamas* (See *sutras*: 2.30, 2.35)

Amaterasu O-mi-kami — the Sun Goddess, represented by the sun, in Japanese Shinto tradition

Ananda — bliss

Aparigraha — non-greed; one of the *yamas* (See *sutras*: 2.30, 2.39)

Asana — steady, comfortable posture; the third of the eight limbs of Ashtanga Yoga (See *sutras*: 2.29, 2.46-48)

Ashram — a spiritual community where seekers practice and study; often associated with a central teacher or guru

Ashtanga Yoga — the Yoga of eight limbs; another name for Raja Yoga (See *sutras*: 2.28-32, 2.35-55; 3.1-3)

Asmita — egoism; identification of the power of the Seer with the instrument of seeing (the body-mind); one of the five *kleshas* (See *sutras*: 2.3, 2.6)

Asteya — non-stealing; one of the *yamas* (See *sutras*: 2.30, 2.37)

Atman — the Self or Spirit

Avidya — ignorance; one of the five *kleshas* (See *sutras*: 2.3, 2.4-5)

Avvaiyar — South Indian woman sage and poet who lived in ancient times; imparted yogic wisdom in her verses

Ayurveda — (lit. scripture of life) one of the Indian systems of medicine

Bhagavad Gita — Hindu scripture in which Lord Krishna gives spiritual teachings to Arjuna on a battlefield; part of the Indian epic, the *Mahabharata*

Bhakta — one who follows the path of Bhakti Yoga; a devotee of God

Bhakti Yoga — the Yoga path of devotion to a form of the Divine

Bhastrika — a vigorous form of *pranayama*, or yogic breathing practice; "bellows breath"

Bhava —attitude that characterizes a specific relationship with the Divine in Bhakti Yoga. Traditionally, they are: *shanta bhava, dasya bhava, sakhya bhava, vatsalya bhava,* and *madhurya bhava*

Bindu — a point or dot representing the manifestation or creation of the universe

Brahma, Lord — God as the Creator in Hindu tradition

Brahmacharya — continence; one of the *yamas* (See *sutras*: 2.30, 2.38)

Brahman — the unmanifest supreme consciousness or God; the Absolute, omnipresent reality

Buddhi — intellect; discriminative aspect of the mind

Caussade, Jean-Pierre de (1675-1751) — French Jesuit priest known for his famous work about spiritual life, *Self-Abandonment to Divine Providence*

Chid — knowledge

Chittavikshepa — distractions of the mind-stuff (See *sutras*: 1.30-31)

Chuang-Tzu (also known as Zhuangzi) — Chinese sage and a founder of Chinese Taoism

Coltrane, Alice (1937-2007) — musician and spiritual teacher known for meditative, mystical sound; student and friend of Swami Satchidananda; became Swamini Turiyasangitananda

Dakshinamurti — (lit. south-faced deity) an aspect of Lord Shiva in which he instructs through silence

Darshan — vision or experience of a divine form or being

Dasya bhava — the Bhakti Yoga attitude, or *bhava*, of the devotee as a servant of God

Dharana — the process of fixing the mind on one point; the beginning of meditation; the sixth of the eight limbs of Ashtanga Yoga (See *sutras*: 2.29; 3.1)

Dharma — duty; righteousness

Dhyana — the steady flow of thought upon one object; the culmination of concentration; the seventh of the eight limbs of Ashtanga Yoga (See *sutras*: 2.29; 3.2)

Dirgha svasam — deep, diaphragmatic breathing in three sequential parts; a form of *pranayama*, or yogic breathing practice

Dogen (1200-1253) — Zen Buddhist master who founded the Soto school of Zen

Donne, John — 17th century English metaphysical poet, lawyer, and priest

Draupadi — in the Hindu tradition, a noble queen who lived in ancient times, known for her faith and surrender to God

Dvesha — aversion to what we find painful; one of the five *kleshas* (See *sutras*: 2.3, 2.8)

Guna — quality, or constituent of nature; three *gunas*: *rajas*, *sattva*, *tamas* (See *sutras*: 1.16; 2.15, 2.18-19; 4.32)

Guru — (lit. remover of darkness) spiritual guide, teacher (See *sutra*: 1.26)

Guru Purnima — annual sacred day on the full moon in July, in which devotees pay homage to their guru; Swami Satchidananda celebrated by honoring all the holy saints and sages

Hafiz — 14th century Persian mystic poet

Hahnemann, Samuel (1755-1843) — founder of the alternative medicine system of homeopathy

Hakuin Ekaku (1686-1768) — Japanese Zen Buddhist master who revitalized the Rinzai school of Zen Buddhism through refocusing on *koan* and meditation practice

Hatha Yoga — the physical aspect of Yoga practice; includes postures (*asanas*), breathing techniques (*pranayama*), cleansing practices (*kriyas*), locks (*bandhas*) and seals (*mudras*) (See *sutras*: 2.29, 2.46-50)

Homa — sacred fire ceremony

Indriya — sense organ; organ of perception (See *sutras*: 2.18, 2.54-55)

Initiation — ceremony marking a new stage in spiritual life, such as receiving a sacred mantra, or admission into a monastic order

Integral Yoga — a synthesis of the six main branches of Yoga: Raja, Hatha, Karma, Bhakti, Jnana, and Japa, as taught by Swami Satchidananda

Ishvara — the supreme cosmic soul; God (See *sutras* 1.23-27)

Ishvara pranidhana — worship of God or surrender to the Divine; one of the *niyamas* (See *sutras*: 1.23, 2.1, 2.32, 2.45)

Japa — concentrated repetition of a mantra or holy name (See *sutras*: 1.27-29)

Japa mala — rosary

Japa Yoga — science of mantra repetition

Jayanti — birth anniversary

168

Jnana Yoga — Yoga path of wisdom based on inquiry into the Self

Jnani — one who follows the Jnana Yoga path

Kapalabhati — (lit. skull shining breath) rapid breathing; a form of *pranayama*, or yogic breathing practice

Karma — action and reaction (See *sutras*: 2.12-14; 4.29-30)

Karma Yoga — performing actions as selfless service without expectation of reward or attachment to the results

Kavacham — armor; protective shield effect produced by vibration of mantra repetition

Keith, Kent — in 1968, wrote the "Paradoxical Commandments," poetic ethical commandments for living selflessly

Klesha — fundamental obstruction or obstacle; basic affliction of the mind; underlying cause of suffering; the five *kleshas*: *avidya, asmita, raga, dvesha, abhinivesa* (See *sutras*: 2.3-2.11, 4.29-30)

Kosha — sheath that surrounds the Spirit or consciousness in an individual; there are five layers: the physical, vital, mental-emotional, intellectual, and bliss.

Krishna, Lord — incarnation of Lord Vishnu; teacher in the *Bhagavad Gita*

Kriya Yoga — according to Sri Patanjali, the three preliminary or practical steps in Yoga: *tapas, svadhyaya,* and *Ishvara pranidhana* (See *sutras*: 2.1-2)

Kriyamana (see *Agami*)

Kundalini Shakti — dormant spiritual energy within each individual, stored at the base of the spine, which flows upward through the body when awakened

Kurozumi Munetada — founder of Kurozumi sect of Shinto faith; lived in 19th century Japan

Laukika sat — relative reality; worldly truth

Lawrence, Brother (c. 1614-1691) — served in a Carmelite monastery as a lay brother; known for his classic text, *The Practice of the Presence of God*

Light Of Truth Universal Shrine (LOTUS) — located at Satchidananda Ashram–Yogaville in Buckingham, Virginia; an interfaith shrine dedicated to the one truth that illumines all faiths, celebrating the unity behind the diversity of all the world faiths

Lila — the play of God; the universe manifesting as the creative activity of God

Madhurya bhava — the Bhakti Yoga attitude, or *bhava*, of the devotee as the lover of the beloved

Magid of Mezeritch — 18th century spiritual leader in the Jewish tradition, who taught the mystical philosophy underlying the teachings of his master, Rabbi Yisrael Baal Shem Tov, who founded Hasidic Judaism

Mahabharata — the great Hindu epic, which includes the *Bhagavad Gita*

Mahasamadhi — (lit. great *samadhi*) the final conscious exit of a realized soul from the physical body

Manas — desiring faculty of the mind; recording faculty of the mind; displays information

Mantra — (lit. that which makes the mind steady) a sound formula for meditation (See *sutras*: 1.27-29)

Maya — power of illusion

Mirabai (1498-1546) — a Hindu saint known for her devotional love songs to Lord Krishna

Nadi suddhi — rhythmic alternate nostril breathing; a form of *pranayama*, or yogic breathing practice

Nama — name

Nasrudin — a 13th century Sufi master who taught through humorous stories

Neti-neti — an analytical technique in which one rejects as unreal everything that is subject to change, as a way of realizing our true nature; "not this, not this"

Niebuhr, Reinhold (1892-1971) — American theologian known for relating Christianity to politics and world affairs; author of the "Serenity Prayer"

Niyama — the five observances; the second of the eight limbs of Ashtanga Yoga (See *sutras*: 2.29, 2.32, 2.40-45)

Non-attachment — Patanjali defines as "the consciousness of self-mastery in one who is free from craving from objects seen or heard about"; supreme non-attachment occurs when, according to Patanjali, "there is non-thirst for even the *gunas* due to realization of the *Purusha* (or true Self)" (See *sutras*: 1.12, 1.15-16)

OM — *pranava*, the cosmic sound vibration which includes all other sounds and vibrations; the basic hum of the universe; the basic mantra; the absolute *Brahman* as sound (See *sutras*: 1.27-28)

Parabhakti — supreme devotion

Parajnanam — supreme wisdom

Paramarthika sat — absolute reality

Patanjali Maharishi —Yogi and sage who compiled the *Yoga Sutras*

Practice — Patanjali defines as "effort toward steadiness of mind" (See *sutras*: 1.12-14; 2.28)

Prakriti — nature; the creation (See *sutras*: 2.17-26)

Prana — vital energy (See *sutras*: 1.34; 2.49)

Pranava — (see *OM*)

Pranayama — the practice of controlling *prana*, usually through control of the breath; the fourth of the eight limbs of Ashtanga Yoga (See *sutras*: 2.29, 2.49-53)

Pranidhana — total dedication

Prarabdha — the karma that has caused one's present birth

Prasad — consecrated offering; divine blessing; grace

Pratipaksha bhavana — practice of substituting opposite thought forms in the mind; replacing a negative thought with an opposite positive one; reflecting on the fact that negative thoughts and actions are based on ignorance and are certain to bring pain (See *sutras*: 2.33-34)

Pratyahara — sense control; withdrawal of the senses from their objects (See *sutras*: 2.29, 2.54-55)

Puja — worship service

Purusha — the divine Self that abides in all things; the true Self (See *sutras*: 1.16, 1.24; 2.6, 2.17-26)

Rabi'a al-'Adawiyya (8th century) — Sufi saint, mystic, and poet known for her holy life and beautiful poems in praise of God as the Beloved

Raga — attachment to what we find pleasurable; one of the five *kleshas* (See *sutras*: 2.3, 2.7)

Raja Yoga — (lit. Royal Yoga) One of the six classical schools of Indian philosophy; set forth in the *Yoga Sutras of Patanjali*; aims at total self-mastery by controlling the mind through meditation; culminates in the highest *samadhi,* or super-conscious state of awareness

Rajas — activity; restlessness; one of the three *gunas*

Rama, Lord — incarnation of Lord Vishnu; a powerful seed mantra

Ramakrishna Paramahamsa (1836-1886) — saint of India, Guru of Swami Vivekananda

Ramana Maharshi (1879-1950) — sage of Tiruvannamalai; spiritual master whose teachings emphasize the Jnana Yoga practice of Self-inquiry

Rig Veda — the earliest of the *Vedas,* the most ancient scriptures of India; consists of over 1000 hymns in praise of the gods

Robert I (Robert the Bruce) (1274-1329) — a heroic king of Scotland who led Scotland in gaining independence from England

Roti — an Indian bread

Rupa — form; appearance

Sadhana — spiritual practice

Sadhana Chatushtaya — a four-fold path of spiritual practice as a means to salvation, which includes discrimination, dispassion, six virtuous qualities, and intense longing for liberation; the six virtuous qualities are: serenity of mind, sense control, withdrawing from desire for sense enjoyment, endurance, faith, and concentration

Sadhu — a spiritual seeker, often a wandering mendicant

Sahaja samadhi — (lit. the easy, natural *samadhi*) a state of *samadhi* in which one retains awareness of supreme peace within while interacting in the world

Sakhya bhava — the Bhakti Yoga attitude, or *bhava*, of regarding God as a beloved friend

Sakshitvam bhavana — identifying with the stable part of the mind that is the witness; watching the thought waves of the mind without attachment

Samadhi — contemplation; super-conscious state; absorption; the eighth and final limb, or culmination of the eight limbs of Ashtanga Yoga (See *sutras*: 2.29; 3.3)

Samsara — repeating cycle of birth, life, death, and rebirth

Samskara — mental impression in the subconscious level of the mind (See *sutra*: 2.15)

Sanchita — karma awaiting another lifetime to bear fruit

Sangha — community of seekers who follow the teachings of a spiritual master or particular spiritual teachings

Sankalpa — a strong resolve

Sankhya — one of the six classical schools of Hindu philosophy; the metaphysics (analysis of reality) it presents provides a framework for the *Yoga Sutras*

Sannyasa — renunciation

Sannyasin — a renunciate; member of the Holy Order of *Sannyas*; a Hindu monk

Santosha — contentment; one of the *niyamas* (See *sutras*: 2.32, 2.42)

Sarasvati — the Goddess of wisdom in the Hindu pantheon

Sari — traditional dress worn by Indian women

Sat — existence or truth

Satchidananda Ashram–Yogaville® — spiritual center, Yoga *ashram,* and community founded by Swami Satchidananda, built on the precepts of Integral Yoga; located in Buckingham, Virginia, USA

Satchidananda, Swami (1914-2002) — revered Yoga master and founder of Integral Yoga, the Integral Yoga Institutes, and Satchidananda Ashram–Yogaville; established the Light Of Truth Universal Shrine (LOTUS) as part of his mission to promote interfaith understanding and harmony

Satsang — (lit. company of the wise) spiritual gathering

Sattva — purity; balanced state; one of the three *gunas*

Satyagraha — a form of non-violent resistance developed by Mahatma Gandhi, which helped gain India's independence from British control

Saucha — purity; one of the *niyamas* (See *sutras*: 2.32, 2.40-41)

Self (see also **Purusha**) — one's true nature (See *sutras*: 1.3-4, 1.16)

Shankaracharya, Adi (788-820) — one of India's greatest philosophers and teachers; proponent of *Advaita Vedanta* philosophy of non-dualism; organized ten monastic orders in India

Shanta bhava — the Bhakti Yoga attitude, or *bhava*, of resting peacefully in God

Shiva, Lord — God as auspiciousness

Shiva Nataraja — Lord Shiva as the Cosmic Dancer; a popular form of God in Hinduism depicting the five functions of the Divine

Shivalingam — a symbol of Lord Shiva

Sivananda, Swami (1887-1963) — renowned sage of the Himalayas; founder of the Divine Life Society; author of hundreds of books on Yoga; Guru of Swami Satchidananda

Sloka — a Sanskrit verse

Steindl-Rast, Br. David (1926-   ) — a Catholic Benedictine monk, pioneer in interfaith dialogue, and teacher of gratefulness as a spiritual practice

Subramuniyaswami, Sivaya (1927-2001) — founder of the Saiva Siddhanta Church and *Hinduism Today* magazine; promoted Hinduism worldwide

Sukha purvaka — rhythmic alternate nostril breathing combined with breath retention; a form of *pranayama*, or yogic breathing practice

Sutra — (lit. thread) aphorism; condensed verse

Svadharma — one's own duty or role to fulfill in life

Svadhyaya — spiritual study; one of the *niyamas* (See *sutras*: 2.1, 2.32, 2.44)

Swami — (lit. master of one's own self); Hindu religious title usually for a *sannyasin*; a term of respect

Tagore, Rabindranath (1861-1941) — Bengali poet and mystic; also an artist, philosopher, playwright, musical composer, and novelist; India's first Nobel Prize recipient, receiving the 1913 Nobel Prize for Literature

Talmud — body of Jewish law and tradition; a key text of Rabbinic Judaism

Tamas — inertia; dullness; one of the three *gunas*

Tao Teh Ching — ancient Taoist scripture

Tapas — (lit. to burn) accepting but not causing pain; accepting pain as help for purification; spiritual austerity; one of the *niyamas* (See *sutras*: 2.1, 2.32, 2.43)

Tathastu — (lit. be it so)

Teresa of Avila (1515-1582) — saint, mystic, and leader in the Catholic Reformation; reformed the Carmelite religious order; wrote many spiritual books on contemplative life

Tirukkural — ancient scripture of South India, authored by the poet, Tiruvalluvar; conveys ethical wisdom through its poetic verses

Upanishads — the final portion of each of the four *Vedas*; present the teachings of *Advaita Vedanta*, exploring the nature of ultimate reality

Vatsalya bhava — the Bhakti Yoga attitude, or *bhava*, in which God is worshipped as one's child

Vedanta — non-dualistic Indian philosophy found in the *Vedas*

Vedas — the most ancient wisdom scriptures of Hinduism (*Rig*, *Sama*, *Yajur*, and *Atharva*)

Venkatesananda, Swami (1921-1982) — spiritual master and sage of practical Yoga wisdom; disciple of Swami Sivananda and brother monk of Swami Satchidananda

Vidyalayam — (lit. temple of learning) school

Vivekananda, Swami (1863-1902) — a disciple of Sri Ramakrishna and one of the founders of the Ramakrishna Order; brilliant teacher and author of many books on Yoga, including his influential commentary on the *Yoga Sutras*

Vritti — mental modification; thought-wave or fluctuation of the mind (See *sutras*: 1.2, 1.4-12)

Wallace Black Elk (1921-2004) — Native American teacher and spiritual leader

Yajna — ritual sacrifice

Yama — the five abstinences; the first of the eight limbs of Ashtanga Yoga (See *sutras*: 2.29-31, 2.35-39)

Yantra — a mystic symbol in the form of a geometric diagram

Yoga — (lit. union) union of the individual with the Absolute; any practice that produces such union; control over the thought waves of the mind; peaceful state of mind under all conditions (See *sutras*: 1.1-3)

Yoga Sutras of Patanjali (see *Raja Yoga*) — a seminal Yoga text of condensed verses by Sri Patanjali Maharishi; the system of Raja Yoga

Yogabrashtas — souls who practiced Yoga in their previous birth, who are reborn into an environment conducive to continuing on the yogic path

Yogananda, Paramahansa (1893-1952) — a spiritual master, whose famed *Autobiography of a Yogi* introduced many Westerners to the science of Yoga

Yudhisthira — a righteous king and eldest of the Pandavas in the Hindu epic, the *Mahabharata*

Bibliography

Caussade, J. P. de, Father. *Self-Abandonment to Divine Providence.* Translated by Algar Thorold. Edited by Father John Joyce, S.J. Rockford: Tan Books and Publishers, Inc., 1987.

Cornell, Joseph. *With Beauty Before Me.* Nevada City: Dawn Publications, 2000.

Feldman, Christina and Kornfield, Jack. *Stories of the Spirit, Stories of the Heart: Parables of the Spiritual Path from Around the World.* New York: HarperSanFrancisco, 1991.

Ladinsky, Daniel. *I Heard God Laughing: Renderings of Hafiz.* Walnut Creek: Sufism Reoriented, 1996.

Lao Tzu. *Lao Tzu: Tao Teh Ching.* Translated by John C. H. Wu. Edited by Paul K. T. Sih. Boston: Shambhala Publications, Inc., 1989.

Lawrence, Brother. *The Practice of the Presence of God.* Translated by Robert J. Edmonson. Edited by Hal M. Helms. Brewster: Paraclete Press, 2010.

Ramakrishna, Sri. *The Gospel of Sri Ramakrishna.* Translated by Swami Nikhilananda. New York: Ramakrishna-Vivekananda Center, 1942.

Satchidananda, Swami. *Meditation: Excerpts from Talks by Sri Swami Satchidananda.* Pomfret Center: Integral Yoga Publications, 1975.

———. *The Living Gita: The Complete Bhagavad Gita.* Buckingham: Integral Yoga Publications, 1988.

———, translation and commentary. *The Yoga Sutras of Patanjali.* Buckingham: Integral Yoga Publications, 2012.

Sivananda, Swami. *Bliss Divine: A Book of Spiritual Essays on the Lofty Purpose of Human Life and the Means to its Achievement.* Uttar Pradesh: Divine Life Society, 1974.

————. *Science of Yoga*, vols. 3 and 5. Uttar Pradesh: Divine Life Society, 1981.

————. *Thought-Power*. 6th ed. Uttar Pradesh: Divine Life Society, 1980.

Smith, Margaret. *Rabi'a The Mystic, A.D. 717 – 801 and Her Fellow Saints in Islam*. San Francisco: The Rainbow Bridge, 1977.

Tiruvalluvar. *The Tirukkural (A Unique Guide to Moral, Material and Spiritual Prosperity)*. Translated by G. Vanmikanathan. Tamilnadu: Tirukkural Prachar Sangh, 1969.

Venkatesananda, Swami, translation and commentary. *The Yoga Sutras of Patanjali*. Uttar Pradesh: Divine Life Society, 1998.

Vivekananda, Swami. *Raja-Yoga*. rev. ed. New York: Ramakrishna-Vivekananda Center, 1982.

About Sri Swami Satchidananda and Integral Yoga

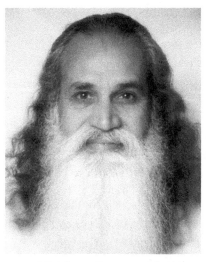

Sri Swami Satchidananda was one of the great Yoga masters to bring the classical Yoga tradition to the West in the 1960s. He taught Yoga postures and meditation, and he introduced students to a vegetarian diet and a more compassionate lifestyle.

During this period of cultural awakening, iconic Pop artist Peter Max and a small circle of his artist friends invited Sri Swamiji to extend an intended two-day visit to New York City so that they could learn from him the secret of attaining physical health, mental peace, and spiritual enlightenment.

Three years later, he led some half a million American youth in chanting *OM*, when he delivered the official opening remarks at the 1969 Woodstock Music and Art Festival and became known as "the Woodstock Guru."

The distinctive teachings he brought with him integrate the physical discipline of Yoga, the spiritual philosophy of India, and the interfaith ideals he pioneered. Those techniques and concepts influenced a generation and spawned a Yoga culture that is flourishing today. Currently, more than twenty million Americans practice Yoga as a means for managing stress, promoting health, slowing down the aging process, and creating a more meaningful life.

The teachings of Swami Satchidananda have entered the mainstream, and there are now thousands of Integral Yoga® teachers around the globe. Integral Yoga Institutes, teaching centers, and certified teachers throughout the United States and abroad offer classes, workshops, retreats, and teacher training programs featuring all aspects of Integral Yoga. Integral Yoga is also the foundation for Dr. Dean Ornish's landmark work in reversing heart disease and Dr. Michael Lerner's noted Commonweal Cancer Help program.

In 1979, Sri Swamiji was inspired to establish Satchidananda Ashram–Yogaville. Founded on his teachings, it is a place where people of different faiths and backgrounds can come to realize their essential oneness. One of the focal points of Yogaville is the Light Of Truth Universal Shrine (LOTUS). This unique interfaith shrine honors the Spirit that unites all the world faiths, while it celebrates their diversity. People from all over the world come there to meditate and pray.

Over the years, Sri Swamiji received many honors for his public service, including the Juliet Hollister Interfaith Award presented at the United Nations and, in 2002, the U Thant Peace Award. On the occasion of his birth centennial in 2014, he was posthumously honored with the James Parks Morton Interfaith Award by the Interfaith Center of New York.

In addition, he served on the advisory boards of many Yoga, world peace, and interfaith organizations. He is the author of numerous books on Yoga and he is the subject of the documentary, *Living Yoga: The Life and Teachings of Swami Satchidananda.*

For more information, visit: www.swamisatchidananda.org and www.yogaville.org.

ABOUT THE AUTHOR

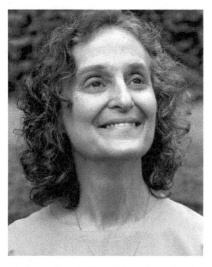

Swami Karunananda is a senior disciple of Sri Swami Satchidananda, the founder of Integral Yoga®, Satchidananda Ashram, and the Integral Yoga Institutes and Centers. With over forty years experience teaching all aspects of Yoga, Swami Karunananda is one of Integral Yoga's master teachers. She specializes in programs that focus on the science of meditation, the philosophy of Yoga, Yoga breathing techniques for better health and well-being, and personal transformation. In 1989, she developed the Integral Yoga Teacher Training course in Raja Yoga and, in 1991, Pranayama and Meditation Teacher Training. She has since conducted many workshops, retreats, and teacher training programs worldwide.

Swami Karunananda compiled and edited the *Lotus Prayer Book,* an interfaith book of prayers, and *Enlightening Tales As Told By Sri Swami Satchidananda.* She was contributing editor for *The Breath of Life: Integral Yoga Pranayama* and for *Integral Yoga® Magazine.* The current volume is an expression of her lifelong love for the study and practice of Yoga.